Mental Health
and
Psychiatric
Nursing

Mental Health and Psychiatric Nursing

K. LALITHA
RN, RM, BSc(PC), MN, PhD
Associate Professor
National Institute of Mental Health
and Neurosciences (NIMHANS)
Bangalore

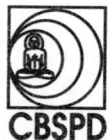

CBSPD

CBS Publishers & Distributors Pvt Ltd

New Delhi • Bengaluru • Chennai • Kochi • Kolkata • Lucknow• Mumbai
Hyderabad • Jharkhand • Nagpur • Patna • Pune • Uttarakhand

Mental Health and
Psychiatric Nursing

ISBN: 978-81-239-1669-9

Copyright © Author and Publisher

First Edition: 1995
Reprint: 1997, 1999, 2000, 2006, 2008
CBS Reprint: 2009, 2024, **2025**

Published by **Satish Kumar Jain** and produced by **Varun Jain** for

CBS Publishers & Distributors Pvt Ltd
4819/XI Prahlad Street, 24 Ansari Road, Daryaganj, New Delhi 110 002, India.
Ph: 011-23266838, 23289259   Website: www.cbspd.com
                                e-mail: delhi@cbspd.com
Corporate Office: 204 FIE, Industrial Area, Patparganj, Delhi 110 092
Ph: 011-4934 4934   Fax: 011-4934 4935
                            e-mail: publishing@cbspd.com; publicity@cbspd.com

Branches

- **Bengaluru:** Seema House 2975, 17th Cross, KR Road, Banasankari 2nd Stage, Bengaluru 560 070, Karnataka, India
  Ph: +91-80-26771678/79   Fax: +91-80-26771680   e-mail: bangalore@cbspd.com
- **Chennai:** 18/8B, Subbarayan Street, Shenoy Nagar, Chennai 600 030, Tamil Nadu, India
  Ph: +91-44-42032115, 26681266   e-mail: chennai@cbspd.com
- **Kochi:** 42/1325, 1326, Power House Road, Opp KSEB, Power House, Ernakulum Kochi 682 018, Kerala, India
  Ph: +91-484-4059061-65,67   Fax: +91-484-4059065   e-mail: kochi@cbspd.com
- **Kolkata:** 147, Hind Ceramics Compound, 1st Floor, Nilgunj Road, Belghoria, Kolkata-700056, West Bengal, India
  Ph: +033-25633055, 033-25633056   e-mail: kolkata@cbspd.com
- **Lucknow:** Basement, Khushnuma Complex, 7 Meerabai Marg (Behind Jawahar Bhawan), Lucknow-226001, UP, India
  Ph: +0522-4000032   e-mail: tiwari.lucknow@cbspd.com
- **Mumbai:** PWD Shed, Gala no 25/26, Ramchandra Bhatt Marg, Next to JJ Hospital Gate no. 2, Opp. Union Bank of India, Noorbaug, Mumbai-400009, Maharashtra, India
  Ph: 022-66661880/89   e-mail: mumbai@cbspd.com

Representatives

• Hyderabad	0-9885175004	• Jharkhand	0-9811541605	• Nagpur	0-8692091830
• Patna	0-9334159340	• Pune	0-9664372571	• Uttarakhand	0-9716462459

Printed at Sanjay Printers, Sahibabad, UP, India

PREFACE

I undertook to write this textbook of Mental Health and Psychiatric Nursing based on the General nursing and midwifery syllabus outlined by Indian Nursing Council (INC, 1986) because of the fact that no nursing personnel has ever made an attempt to write a book. Surprisingly enough, there are very few texts (three or four) in psychiatric nursing field, written by nursing personnel in India, relate to the specific psychiatric conditions and peculiarities of psychiatry. Instead the book systematically deals with the topics prescribed by INC for the nursing students of General nursing and midwifery programme.

Psychiatric nursing practice and education have gone through many changes in the past decade, and with these changes comes the need to make understandable and meaningful information accessible to nurses and students. Unlike other text books that attempt to cover every aspect of psychiatric nursing and that superficially cover many important topics, this book focuses on the practical, essential information that General Nursing students need to effectively care for patients and successfully interact with other members of the health care team.

Mental Health and Psychiatric Nursing text takes a practical, clinical approach to nursing, integrating clinical realities with the theory taught in Schools of Nursing and emphasizing those duties for which nurses primarily are responsible.

The text is organised in six units. Unit one, Introduction and Review, explores the meaning of mental illness, concept of mental health and reviews mental mechanisms.

Unit two deals with the evolution of psychiatry, and oetiology of mental illness and the contributing factors of mental illness. It also gives introductory note about the legal aspects in the care of the mentally sick.

Community responsibility towards mentally ill, attitude and misconception of people towards mentally ill are presented in the third unit. Health and social services that are available in the community for the mentally sick is also dealt in detail in this unit.

The unit four focuses on the various approaches used for making diagnosis of mentally ill individuals. The unit opens with the general discussion on early recognition of deviations from the normal, followed by conceptual models to explain the deviated patterns of behaviour/ abnormal behaviour from normal. This unit specifically focuses on the physical, psychological and social functions disturbances seen in mentally ill individuals. This unit also incorporates the latest systems of classification, namely ICD-10 and Indian classification of mental illness for easy understanding. The last part of this unit discusses about signs and symptoms of common mental illnesses.

Unit five contains eleven chapters devoted to management of psychiatric patients in the hospitals and in the community. They are mainly drug therapy, physical therapy and psychotherapy. It also deals with topics like hypnosis, narcoanalysis and psychoanalysis. The chapter on behaviour therapy discusses the various techniques adopted to modify the sick behaviour of psychiatric patients. The main aspect of psychiatric nursing in occupational, recreational and social therapy are explained in detail. The chapter on legal aspects of psychiatric nursing describes the legal implications involved in psychiatric nursing practice, civil rights and criminal responsibilities of the mentally ill person. The unit concludes with the chapter on rehabilitation of mentally restored patients. It highlights on acceptance and non-acceptance of the cured patient by family and community, and the various problems faced by patients for rehabilitative services. It stresses on different therapeutic approaches that could be employed by nurses to rehabilitate the patient in terms of re-employment and follow-up.

Unit six, the last unit of the book, has seven chapters deals with the role of nurses in hospital and in community with special emphasis on National Mental Health Program for India (NMHP). This unit also addresses the nurses to have specific attitudes towards the mentally ill, basic needs of patients and the sharpened focus on the principles of psychiatric nursing. It presents a refined analysis of American Standards of Psychiatric Nursing in Indian Context. Chapters on ways of meeting aggression and violent behaviour present the psychodynamics, phases and nursing care of those patients with specific guide lines based on nursing goals and interventions. The next two chapters deal with nursing management of patients diagnosed as withdrawal, mania and depression. They critically analyse the psychodynamics, bio-psychosocial and nursing management. The chapter on prevention of accidents amongst the mentally ill describes the accident prone situations in the hospitals and in the community and how to prevent them. The chapter on observation, reporting and recording extensively deals with the nurses role in it.

The last chapter of the unit deals with the legal aspects of the care of mentally sick patients. It describes the salient features of Indian Lunacy Act, 1912 and also the Mental Health Act, 1987.

The text book has the most current material in the field of mental health and psychiatric nursing. At the end of each chapter simple study questions are placed as a part of learning exercise and to enhance self-evaluation of readers.

With students in mind, I have provided a number of tools to facilitate understanding and promote clinical competence.

- Psychotherapeutic management of patient and specific guidelines to develop individualised care plans for the patients.

- ICD-10 classification of behaviour disorders.

- A glossary for each psychiatric term as and when it appears in the text.

The book also extensively deals with certain chapters such as, Diagnosis, Classification of mental disorders, Drug therapy, Shock therapy, Psychotherapy, Psychoanalysis, Behaviour therapy, Recreational and social therapy, Occupational therapy, Rehabilitation, Legal aspects in psychiatric nursing, Role of nurse in Community Mental Health Nursing, NMHP, Observation, Reporting and recording, etc. to help not only the students of General Nursing, but also those studying for B.Sc., Post-certificate B.Sc. and M.Sc. in psychiatric nursing programs. It will also be helpful to the nursing teachers.

As this text book on Mental Health - Psychiatric Nursing goes to print, I am content that I have maintained and furthered the quality of writing, content, meaning and usefulness. I am proud of the result, and hope that it will continue to interest and inspire readers to explore the challenges of mental health and psychiatric nursing.

Finally, thanks are also due to M/s. Gajanana Book Publishers and Distributors, for undertaking this publication, thus fulfilling a long time requirement of an excellent book on Mental Health and Psychiatric Nursing. I also thank M/s. Typograph for typesetting and graphic work.

Bangalore   K. Lalitha

Date:16-1-1995

CONTENTS

Legal aspects of psychiatric nursing Rehabilitation
- acceptance of the cured patient
by the family and the community
- re-employment
- follow up

UNIT-VI Role of the Nurses

The role of the nurses in
hospital and community
in psychiatric nursing :-

Attitude to mental illness
- Adaptation required in meeting
basic and nursing needs
- Ways of meeting aggression and
violent behaviour
- Depression
- Withdrawal and mania
- Prevention of accidents amongst
mantally ill
- Observation reporting and recording

Legal aspects of the care of mentally

sick patients
- Procedure for admission into and
discharge from mental hospitals.

INTRODUCTION AND REVIEW

Meaning of mental illness

Precise definitions of mental illness or disorder are impractical. Many define mental illness as "psychiatric disease" or "behaviour disorder". While explaining, they say that "person expresses his mental distress through thought, feelings and actions".

Disturbances seen in behaviour are named as mental illness. To define behaviour, everything that organism does from the day of conception till death is called behaviour. That everything includes,

Knowing   – Cognative   – Thinkingor
                                     thought processes

Feeling   – Affective   – Emotions

Doing   – Conative   – Action or psycho
                                     motor activities

An individual either showing all the three areas of disturbances like flight of ideas, (ideas fly from one

1

topic to another as thinking disturbances) euphoria (feeling excessively happy as emotional disturbance) and withdrawal (motor retardation as action disturbances) or either one of the areas being disturbed is called as mentally ill.

For example, a patient who is diagnosed as having mania, has the behaviour disturbances of thinking, feeling and doing. Manic patients have euphoria, flight of ideas and excessive psycho-motor activities. Patients with Schizophrenia, predominantly suffer from cognitive disturbances, namely attention, perception, judgement and thinking.

Outcome of these disturbances, the mental illnesses are identified with the following criteria :

- Dissatisfaction with one's characteristics, abilities and accomplishments.
- Ineffective or unsatisfying interpersonal relationships.
- Dissatisfaction with one's place in the world.
- Ineffective coping or adaptation to the events in one's life as well as a lack of personal growth.
- Inability to communicate with others.

Defining clearly what constitutes mental illness and mental health is not easy.

Review of mental health

Defining health and disease is difficult, since the concepts of both constantly undergo change and development. It is usually much simpler to identify the extremely healthy and the extremely sick than to dis-

2

tinguish between the borderlines of either physical or mental health. The W.H.O definition of health also says that the absence of disease is no longer an acceptable definition of health in either the physical or the emotional sense.

Mental health is much more difficult to define than mental illness. Many experts who have attempted to clarify the concept of Mental health, they emphasised one aspect or another of what they consider to be mental health. One of the few studies to examine mental health reported six dimensions to evaluate mental health. They were : unhappiness, lack of gratification, strain, feelings of vulnerability, lack of self-confidence, and uncertainty. Yet problems still exist in the definition of mental health.

Mental health is often spoken of as a state of well-being such as happiness, contentment, satisfaction or achievement. Happiness is a desirable consequence of mental health, but it cannot be used as a criterion. In a state of mental health, the person functions comfortably within his society and is satisfied with himself and his achievements.

We say that someone is mentally healthy when we observe in the person a balance between the integrated body, mind, and spirit and the environment. The fact is, though, that no generally accepted definition of mental health exists. Rather, we infer the presence or absence of mental health from an individual's behaviour.

Mental health implies mastery in the areas of life involving love, work and play. After an extensive survey of literature, Marie Jahoda indicated six general approaches used to develop criteria for the existence or absence of mental health. These include :

- positive attitudes towards self
- growth, development and self-actualisation
- integration
- autonomy
- adequate contact with reality

- environmental mastery

Positive attitudes towards self

It includes an acceptance of self and self-awareness. An individual must have confidence on his own self, and positive opinion on his ability. He must also have a sense of identity, a wholeness, belongingness, security and meaningfulness. He must have a goal in life and must put effort constantly to achieve it. The goal accomplishment further strengthens his positive attitudes towards self.

Growth, development and self-actualisation

Maslow and Rogers developed extensive theories on the development and realisation of the human potential. Maslow describes the concept of "self-actualisation" and Rogers emphasises the "fully functioning person". Both theories focus on the entire range of human adjustment. They describe a self engaged in a constant quest, always seeking new growth, develoment and challenges. These theories focus on the total person and whether:

- he is adequately in touch with his own self to free the resources that are there. In other words, the person is willing to depart from the status quo to progress towards self-realisation and maximisation of his capacities;

4

- he has free access to his feelings and can integrate them with his intellectual and cognitive functioning;
- he is effective, competent and able to interact freely and openly with others;
- he can share himself with other people and grow from such experiences.

Integration

It is a balance between what is expressed and what is repressed, between outer and inner conflicts and drives, and a regulation of one's moods and emotions. It includes emotional responsiveness and control and a unified philosophy of life. This consistent set of values provides a framework for continuity in all responses. This criterion can be measured at least in past by the person's ability to withstand stress and cope with anxiety. A strong ego enables the person to handle change and grow from it.

Autonomy

It involves self-determination, a balance between dependence and independence, and acceptance of the consequences of one's actions. It implies that the person is responsible for himself, including his decisions, actions, thoughts and feelings. Consequently, the person demonstrates autonomy, a sense of detachment, independence and a tendency to look within for guiding values and rules to live by. He acts independently, dependently or interdependently as the need arises, without permanently losing his independence. This self-governance makes the person to respect autonomy and freedom in others.

Adequate contact with reality

The person distinguishes fact from fantasy, the real world from a dream world, and acts accordingly. In otherword, reality perception is the individual's ability to test his assumptions about the world by empirical thought. The mentally healthy person can change his perceptions in the light of new information. This criterion includes empathy or social sensitivity, a respect for the feelings and attitudes of others.

Environmental mastery

It enables a mentally healthy person to feel success in an approved role in his society or group. He can deal effectively with the world, work out his problems of living, and obtain satisfaction from life. This criterion incorporates the idea of social competence as well. The person should be able to cope with loneliness, aggression, and frustration without being overwhelmed. The mentally healthy person can respond to others, love and be loved and cope with reciprocal relationships. He can build new friendships and have satisfactory social group involvement.

Evidence of mental health is usually seen in a person's meaningful work, enjoyment of life, humour, ability to benefit from rest and sleep, optimism, spontaneity, satisfying relationships with others, ability to work well alone and with others, sound judgement and decisions, acceptance of responsibility for actions, ability to give and receive, behaviour that is generally accepted by the group, and direct expressions of emotions, including strong feelings.

Finally, a person should not be assessed against some vague or ideal notion of health. Rather, he should be seen in a group context, an age context and an individual context. The issue is not how well someone fits an arbitrary age standard, but rather what is reasonable for a particular person. Such a view incorporates the concept of individual's coping or adjustment ability. This dimension equates mental health with adaptation and mental illness with maladaptation.

Adaptation ability and the nature varies from individual to individual. They are based on biological, socio-cultural or psychological factors. Biological factors include prenatal, perinatal, physique, neuro anatomy and physiology. Socio-cultural factors are family stability, child rearing patterns, economic level, housing, membership in a minority that may experience the effects of prejudice or inadequate health resources, religious influences, and values. Psychological factors are parent and sibling-infant/child interactions, intelligence quotient (IQ), self-concept, skills, talents, creativity and emotional development level.

Review of mental mechanisms

Mental mechanisms are also referred to as ego-defense mechanisms, coping mechanisms and defense mechanisms. Mental mechanisms function to protect the ego from overwhelming anxiety; for the most part, they operate on an unconscious level. They are the patterns of adjustment through which an individual relieves or decreases anxiety caused by an uncomfortable situation that threatens self-esteem.

As we consider adaptation/adjustment as a sign of mental health and maladaptation/maladjustment as a sign of mental illness, mental mechanisms are patterns of adjustment. It is necessary to know what adjustment is.

7

Adjustment is the process by which an individual maintains a balance between its needs and the circumstances that influence the satisfaction of these needs.

Adjustment process can be described by the pattern shown in figure 1 and 2.

A nursing student has a goal of getting success in her examination. When she passes through her examination with first class she feels highly satisfied and her internal environment is   full with joy, contentment and feelings competence.

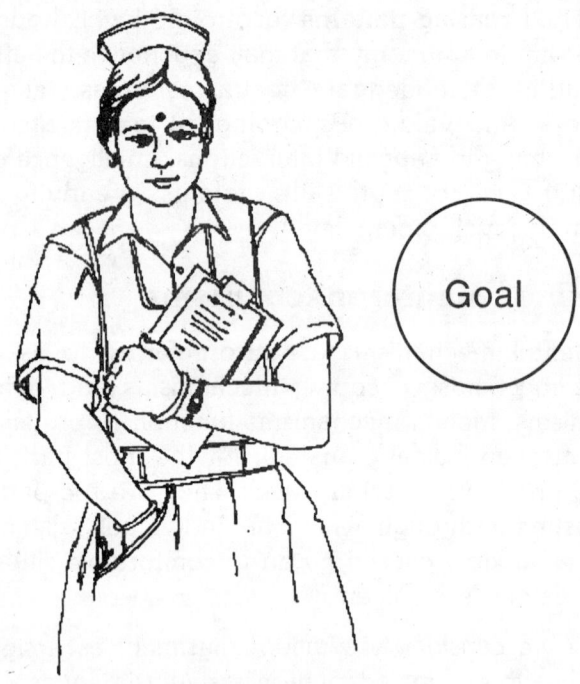

Figure 1

In case the same student gets obstacles like medical illness, sad news from home, or language problem to understand the subjects which lead to delay in achieving her goal in the life, she may not be passing her examination in one attempt. The delay in meeting her goal may result in a variety of physical and emotional disorders such as migraine, headaches, peptic ulcers, myocardial infarctions ("heart attacks"), hypertension, suicide, mental illness and the feelings of "hopelessness" and "unhappiness". This disturbed internal homeostasis or delay in achieving the goal brings out various adjustment responses in her. (See Figure 2)

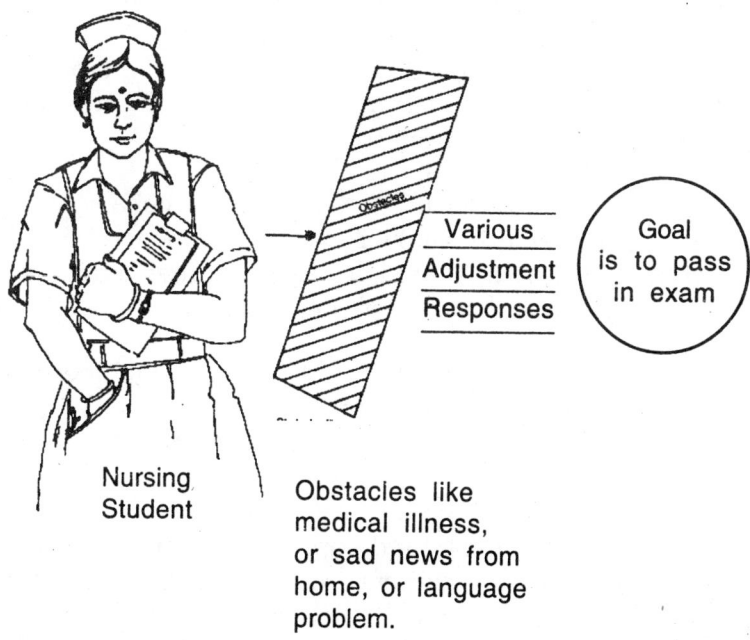

Nursing Student

Obstacles like medical illness, or sad news from home, or language problem.

Figure 2. Adjustment process

These adjustment responses are mental mechanisms. They protect one's ego from overwhelming anxiety; for the most part, they operate on an unconscious level.

Similarly when an individual faces the stressful life events, he adapts to the situation with his mental mechanisms. The nature of mechanism that she chooses is based upon her life experience of having used a mechanism successfully or not, role model and the pre-disposed ability. The success in using the mechanism strengthens her problem solving ability and adds to the learning experience in the life. The failure in mental mechanism becomes a potential health problem. She starts using the inappropriate mental mechanisms too frequently and fails to achieve her goal and comes out with maladaptive responses like Neurotic health problems (such as anxiety, reactive depression & phobia etc.) or psychotic health problems (depression, paranoid schizophrenia)

Hence we understand that nature of behaviour of any human being is partly depended upon the type of mental mechanism is used to adapt to a situation, as a response to the increased demand.

Now let us see the various types of mental mechanisms that are often used by us.

Denial

It is a commonly used coping mechanism wherein a person denies the existence of some external reality. The person using denial is unaware that he is using it. When a patient is informed of his medical diagnosis for example, he usually denies its existence for some period of time.

"Oh no, this is a mistake".

"It's not true".

"There's nothing wrong with me".

There are varying degrees of denial. A person who has been told that he has had a heart attack, which causes a great deal of damage to the heart muscle, may deny that he has had a heart attack at all and say, "I can't have heart attack, I'm too young and healthy".

Another person facing the same diagnosis may acknowledge that he has suffered a heart attack and recognise the need for treatment and for modification of his life style, but may not believe that the extent of heart damage is as serious as his doctors have described.

For a brief or lengthy period of time, denial generally operates as a protective and often a healthy mechanism, protecting the individual from the shock of reality until he is more able to deal with it.

Regression

Through the use of regression, a person avoids anxiety by returning to an earlier, more comfortable time in his life.

A 3-year-old child might regress in response to the birth of a sibling and begin again to soil her garments, suck her thumb, or talk "baby talk" to bring her parental attention. An adult undergoing any physical or emotional stress might reggress by becoming irritable and demanding, or might take to his bed, for a "sick day", thereby giving up his responsibilities for the day and allowing others to meet his needs.

Like the other mental mechanisms regression may be useful and healthy response to stresses, but may become maladaptive if used excessively or exclusively.

Displacement

It is the transfer of an emotion from its original object to a substitute object. For example, if a person is angry with his superior at work or school, he may feel too threatened to confront that individual with his anger; instead he may go home and vent his feelings (anger) from his original object (his superior) to a substitute object (a family member).

It is likely that the individual who displaces his feelings has no awareness that he is using displacement. Later, however, he may look back on the events and realise that, because he was angry with someone to whom he could not comfortably express his feelings, he "took it out" on a member of his family.

Projection

Placing blame for difficulties upon others or attributing one's own unethical desires to others. Others are seen as responsible for one's own short comings, mistakes and misdeeds; and others are seen as responsible for one's unacceptable impulses, thoughts and desires.

For example, the student who fails in her examination may feel that the teacher was unfair; the delinquent teenager may attribute her problems on a rejecting and non understanding parents.

Individuals with paranoid behaviour frequently overuse the mechanism of projection. If the person is fearful of his environment, he may project those feelings on to the external world and develop the delusion that forces in the environment as someone is trying 'to get him'. He may believe that others are constantly watching him and plotting his demise.

Sometimes, projection of feelings functions as an adaptive mechanism, protecting the individuals from feelings that he finds unacceptable to himself until he learns to own up to them and acknowledge them as part of humanity.

Rationalisation

It is the substitution of acceptable reasons for the real or actual reasons motivating behaviour. Through rationalisation, a person justifies his behaviour or conceals his disappointments. For example, if a person interviews for a job but not got selected, he may rationalise that the interviewer did not spend enough time with him to get a fair impression of his strengths. He may also rationalise that he did not really want the job or that the job would have required more time than he was willing to devote to it. In each of these rationalisations, the person covers his real feelings of failure and disappointment with ones that will protect him from the anxiety associated with failure and disappointment.

Repression

It is often referred to as "selective forgetting". Through repression, an individual forces certain feelings or thoughts into his unconscious. The repressed material, such as painful memories or feelings, remain in the person's unconscious, although it may surface from time to time in his dreams or "slips of the tongue". Repression is a mechanism that occurs at the unconscious level.

A student who is caught for her malpractice by the invigilator in the examination hall while writing her examination may find the experience as terribly painful that she excludes it from consciousness and becomes 'amnesic' with regard to the guilty experience.

The usefulness of repression, again, is to protect the individual from overwhelming anxiety. He involuntarily 'forgets' certain events or feelings that evoke a great deal of anxiety.

Suppression

It takes place when a person consciously excludes certain thoughts or feelings from his mind. The excluded thoughts or feelings are those that cause him anxiety. This mental mechanism operates at the conscious level. When a person decides to "put something out of his mind" or "not worry about it until tomorrow", he is using suppression.

A student was assigned a major research paper to write. Everytime she thought about the length and depth of the paper and the amount of hardwork it would require, she felt extremely anxious.

To overcome her anxiety and initiate work on the paper, she decided she would not think about it as a total, completed project, but would break it down into smaller, more manageable units, and then proceeded to tackle each component systematically.

When her anxiety surfaced from time to time, she forced herself to push aside fears about the total understanding and concentrate on the smaller unit of work before her.

Compensation

Compensation is a defense against feelings of inferiority and inadequacy growing out of real or imagined personal defects or weaknesses, as well as out of the individuals inevitable failures and set backs. Compensation mechanism is constructive and deliberate behaviour. For example, an individual who is physically handicapped, through his increased effort may develop an exceptionally pleasing personality. He attempts to substitute for the defect in some way or other to draw attention away from it.

Some compensation mechanisms are unhealthy. For example, the person who feels unloved and frustrated may eat too much. In extreme cases, an individual may engage in anti-social behaviour in an unconscious attempt to get some concern from others.

Sublimation

Sublimation is the mechanism by which a primitive or unacceptable tendency is redirected into socially constructive channels. Individual selects substitutes satisfaction that is healthy. For example it is often assumed that creativeness in the arts is a sublimation of sex motives. A panchayat board president who happens to be a widower, cannot satisfy his sex needs by having extra marital relationships as it would bring down his image in the village. Therefore he selects substitute satisfaction means by displaying nude pictures, statues in and around his house in the name of artistic taste.

Fantasy

Fantasy is a process of gratifying frustrated desires by imaginary achievements. Fantasy is also a non-rational mental activity that allows an individual to escape from his daily pressures and responsibilities. For example, if a person is overwhelmed by the pressures of a task he has undertaken, he may imagine the completion of the task and the feelings of satisfaction and pride he will experience at its completion. These feelings may assist him on to work harder towards his goal.

The excessive use of fantasy, on the other hand, reduces an individual's contact with reality and may render him incapable of dealing with the demands of his life.

The usefulness of these various mental mechanisms lies in their protection of the person from anxiety. We all use these mechanisms at one time or another, particularly in situations that elicit threatening or painful feelings; however, their value depends on their judicious use. The continuous exclusive use of these mechanisms would inhibit or prevent the person from learning other, more effective ways to cope with, adapt to and grow in relation to his environment.

Questions

1. Define behaviour.
2. List six criteria for defining mental health.
3. What is mental mechanism?
4. Explain the process of adjustment.
5. Name the common mental mechanisms and explain each one of them in detail.

MENTAL ILLNESS

History and trends in care

Historically, mental illness was viewed as demonic possession, the influence of ancestral spirits, the result of violating a taboo or neglecting a cultural ritual, and spiritual condemnation. The mentally ill have been rediculed, neglected, banned, persecuted and deprived of their freedoms.

The common belief that mental disturbance was related to super natural phenomena meant that healing, if it were to take place at all, must involve supernatural intercession.

During 11 B.C. Saul King of Israel was found to suffer from manic depressive episodes. During the attack of mania, he stripped off all his clothes in a public place, on other occasions he tried to kill his son Jonathan.

Cambyses, King of Persia during 16th B.C. was one of the first alcoholics on record. When his alcohol consumption was excess, his behaviour was uncontrollable, during which he behaved as a mad man.

George III of England, known as the 'Mad Monarch' showed variety of symptoms, over active and excitement.

The French philosopher Rousseau developed paranoid symptoms during later part of his life. He was obsessed with fear of secret enemies.

The mental disorders in early writings of the Chinese, Egyptians and Greeks shows that mental disorder was caused by demons. They were treated with

- Exorcism   (prayer, noise making and preparation of a purgative made from sheep's dung and wine to be drunk by patient)

- Operation trephining   (trephine is a circular opening made on the skull with crude stone instrument for the evil spirit to escape from the brain.)

Hippocrates (460 B.C.), the great Greek physician, called as "The Father of Model Medicine", emphasised that the mental illness were due to brain pathology. He further classified mental illness into three categories, Mania, Melancholia and Phrenitis. The method of treatment for hysteria was Exorcism. Hippocrates recommended marriage as a treatment for mental illness.

Plato (429 B.C), the great philosopher, believed that mental disorder was partly due to organic, partly due to moral and partly divine. He made provisions of treatment for the mentally ill in the community. He insisted on humane treatment of mentally ill.

He advocated that the mentally disturbed individuals who commit crime are not responsible for the act.

Aristotile (384 B.C), another Greek philosopher, emphasised on the release of repressed emotions for the effective treatment of mental illness. He suggested cathersis and music therapy for patients with Melancholia. He also followed the theory of Hippocrates about the bile disturbances in mentally ill. They believed that the bile is responsible for suicidal impulses.

The earlier concept of Chinese about mentally ill was that the person suffering from excitement, initially feels sadness and sleeplessness. He then be-comes grandiose, feeling that he is great and very noble. Later starts scolding day and night, singing, seeing strange things, hearing strange voices. Chinese views of treatment were more of natural than the super-natural. They withheld the suggested food of patients.

Emergence of humanitarian approach was found when Parcelsus (16th century) insisted that the dancing mania was not a possession, but a form of disease and should be treated.

Zil Boorg and Henry also postulated a conflict between instinctual and spiritual nature of man as a cause for mental illness. This psychological nature of cause for mental illness changed the views about mental illness greatly.

In the 19th century, mental illness was viewed as incurable and little, if any, humane treatment existed. Until 1820, the mentally ill were exhibited, for a fee, as diversion and entertainment for the public. Until 1886, the mentally ill were restrained in iron manacles.

Beginning in the 1950's, pharmacotherapy changed the picture of mental health care. The publication of Sigmond Freud led to new concepts in the treatment of mentally ill. The late 1930's and early 1940's saw the introduction of two empirical treatments - insulin coma therapy and electric shock treatment. Then came the tranquilisers; they made it possible to admit and treat all types of mental illness in the general hospital. The idea that the mental illness patients can be admitted and treated in a general hospital developed. The current trend is complete integration of the mentally ill patient into the normal pattern of medical care with continuity of care from his family doctor, utilisation of the general hospital and community resources.

Surveys of mental morbidity carried out in various parts of India suggest a morbidity rate of not less than 18-20 per 1000 and the types of illness and their prevalence are very much the same as in other parts of the world. At least 10-20 per 1000 suffer from severe mental illness at any given time (requiring urgent care) and at least 3 to 5 times that number suffer from other forms of distressing and socio-economically incapacitating emotional disorders.

Before Independence, the approach in India for the care of the mentally ill person was largely concentrated to build 'asylums'. In 1946, the Bhore Committee presented the situation in regard to mental health services as, "even if the proportion of mental patients be taken as 2 per 1000 population in India, hospital accommodation should be available for atleast 8 lakh patients as against the existing provision for a little over 10,000 beds for the country as a whole". In India, the existing number of mental hospital beds is in the ratio of one bed to about 40,000 of the population. As a follow-up of Bhore committee recommendations, 5 mental hospitals, were set up - Amritsar (1947), Hyderabad (1953), Srinagar (1958), Jama Nagar (1960) and Delhi (1966). An All India Institute of Mental Health, on the recommendations of this committee was set up at Bangalore. (Now it is renamed as National Institute of Mental Health and Neuro Sciences).

In 1978, Alma-Ata Declaration of "Health For All by 2000 A.D." (HFA by 2000 A.D.) brought a major challenge to Indian mental health professional in which India is one of the country to envisage the goal of `HFA by 2000 A.D'. Hence to achieve mental health for all, Government of India, in 1980, called experts to assess the mental health needs and requirements. They brought out National Mental Health Policy for India.

In 1981, at Raipur Rani, Chandigarh and at Sakalwara, Bangalore, a community psychiatric model was set up to experiment primary mental health care approach.

In 1982, Central Council of Health, India's highest health policy making body accepted the National Mental Health Policy and brought out National Mental Health Program for India. Its objectives are,

i) Basic mental health care to all the needy especially the poor from rural, slum and tribal areas.

ii) Application of mental health knowledge in general health care and in social development.

iii) Promote community participation in the men tal health services development and to stimu late efforts towards self-help in the community.

21

The above objectives are expected to be achieved through the following approaches,

i) Integration of the mental health care services with the existing general health services.

ii) To utilise the existing infrastructure of health services and also to deliver the minimum mental health care services.

iii) To provide appropriate task-oriented training to the existing health staff.

iv) To link mental health services with the existing community development program.

In 1990, Government of India formed an 'Action Group' at Delhi to pool the opinions of Mental Health experts about National Mental Health Program. National Institute of Mental Health and Neuro Science, Bangalore has taken up the leadership in orienting the health care professional about mental health programs of our country.

Etiology of mental illness and contributing factors

Etiology is the study of the causes of disease. In psychiatry, the study of causation of mental illness was explained through humoral, demonic and physical theories in the past. But in the last few decades number of theories have been elaborated to explain psychiatric disorders on a scientific basis. Some of the important theories are,

i) Genetic theories

ii) Biochemical theories

iii) Psychological theories

iv) Behavioural and cognitive theories

v) Social theories.

In psychiatry, the study of causation is complicated by two problems. The first problem is that causes are often remote in time from the effects they produce. For example, it is widely believed that childhood experiences partly determine the occurance of neuroses in adult life. It is difficult to test this idea because the necessary information can only be gathered either by studying children and tracing them many years later, which is difficult; or by asking adults about their childhood experiences, which is unreliable.

The second problem is that a **single cause** may lead to **several effects.** For example, deprivation of parental affection in childhood has been reported to predispose an individual to antisocial behaviour, suicide, depressive disorder and several other disorders. Conversely a **single effect** may arise from **several causes.** The later can be illustrated either by different causes in different individuals, or by multiple causes in a single individual. For example, mental handicap/mental retardation (single effect) may occur in one individual through a combination of causes, such as genetic factors, adverse childhood experiences (psychological factor) and stressful events like earthquake, flood or poverty (social factors) in adult life.

A single psychiatric disorder, as just explained, may result from several causes. For this reason, a scheme for classifying cause is required. A useful approach is to divide causes chronologically into pre-disposing, precipitating and perpetuating.

Predisposing factors

These factors determine an individual's susceptibility to mental illness. These predisposing factors interact with precipitating factors to result in mental illness. These are factors, many of them operating from early life, that determine a person's vulnerability to causes acting close to the time of the illness. They include genetic endowment and the environment in utero, as well as physical, psychological and social factors in infancy and early childhood.

Genetic factors

Structural abnormalities in chromosomes cause mental disease. In psychiatry the most important example concerns Down's Syndrome (mongolism). In this condition two kinds of abnormality have been detected: in the first kind there is an additional chromosome (trisomy); in the second kind the chromosome number is normal, but one chromosome is unusually large because a segment of another chromosome is attached to it (translocation).

In family risk studies the investigator determines the risk of a psychiatric condition among the relatives of affected persons, and compares it with the expected risk in the general population. It was found that parents, siblings and children of severely depressed patients have a morbid risk of 10-15 percent for affective disorders, as against 1-2 percent in the general population.

Twin studies suggest that the concordance rates for manic-depressive psychosis were 68 percent for monozygotic twins and 23 percent for dizygotic twins. Similar findings were seen in schizophrenia.

Biological factors

These factors can be directed either to the causes of disease, or to the mechanisms by which disease produces its effects. Eg. : Heredity, constitution, endocrinal, metabolic and biochemical abnormalities, physical defects, illnesses etc.

Psychological factors

The psychological approach to psychiatric etiology is widely supposed that early experiences play an important part in the development of neurosis and psychosis in adult life.

Personality type, temperament, abnormal parent-child relationship, and psychologically traumatic experiences during childhood, preadolescence and adolescence are considered to be causative factors of mental illness.

Psychodynamic theories explain the causation of functional psychosis namely Schizophrenia as follows:

According to Freud, in the first stage of psychological development libido was withdrawn from external objects and attached to the ego. The result was exaggerated self-importance. Since the withdrawal of libido made the external world meaningless, the patient attempted to restore meaning by developing abnormal beliefs. Because of libidinal withdrawal, the Schizophrenic patient could not form a transference, and therefore could not be treated by psycho analysis.

Melanie Klein believed that the origins of Schizophrenia were in infancy. In the 'paranoid-schizoid position' the infant was thought to deal with innate aggressive impulses by splitting both his own ego and his representation of his mother into two incompatible parts, one wholly bad and the other wholly good. Only later did the child realise that the same person could be good at one time and bad at another. Failure to pass through this stage adequately was the basis for the later development of Schizophrenia.

Precipitating factors

These are events that occur shortly before the onset of a disorder and appear to have induced it. They may be again physical, physiological, psychological or social. Whether they produce a disorder at all, and what kind of disorder, depends partly on the constitutional factors of the patient.

Physical factors

They include cerebral tumours or drug intoxication leading to brain dysfunction. That may precipitate a mental illness in vulnerable or predisposed individuals.

Physiological factors

Pregnancy, child birth, menopause, puberty, involution, fever, etc. may be perceived as stress by an individual which in turn precipitates mental illness.

Psychological factors

It includes factors like strained interpersonal relationship, family and marital disharmony, sexual mal-adjustments, or death of a loved one. Sometime the same factor can act in more than one way; for example, a head injury can induce psychological disorder either through physical changes in the brain or through its stressful implications to the patient.

Social factors

The precipitants include change in the life pattern due to environmental factors like earthquake, flood and epidemic attack of contagious diseases may lead to mental illness. Political upheavals and social crises, occupational and financial difficulties owing to poverty, etc. are also considered to be causes of mental illness.

Perpetuating factors

These factors prolong the course of a disorder after it has been provoked. When planning treatment, it is particularly important to give attention to these factors. The original predisposing and precipitating factors may have ceased to act by the time the patient is seen, but the perpetuating factors may well be treatable. For example, patient with alcoholism might have had marital disharmony as pre-disposing factor and got treated for alcoholism but the marital disharmony continue to remain as a cause for further mental illness.

Legal aspects in the care of the mentally sick

Both psychiatry and law deal with human behaviour. Law addresses the outcome of behaviour and has developed a system of rules and regulations to facilitate orderly social functioning. The practice of psychiatry is influenced by the law, particularly in its concern for the rights of patients and the quality of care they are receiving.

The legal aspects of psychiatry in India are based on the Indian Lunacy Act of 1912. According to the Indian Lunacy Act, a mental patient is referred to as a lunatic which is defined as an idiot or a person of unsound mind. A mental hospital is referred to as an asylum established or licensed by the Government to take care of the lunatics.

Indian Lunacy Act of 1912 was revised and the new act was enacted as The Mental Health Act in 1987. This Act, unlike the Indian Lunacy Act of 1912, recognises the crucial role of treatment and care of mentally ill persons. In addition, it also incorporates the newer knowledge and recent concepts in the field of mental health. The basic objective of the Mental Health Act (1987) is not only to discard the outdated concepts of custodial care and segregation of mental patients' from the community, but also to incorporate better provisions relating to treatment and care. For the first time, it brings out judicial safeguards for patients' rights. To prevent any indignity or cruelty to the mentally ill, it introduces humanitarian considerations. There is an explicit protection of their human rights. It also incorporates penalties for establishments and maintenance of mental hospitals/ psychiatric nursing homes in contravention of rules provided in the Act.

In the historical perspective, it is interesting to note that before the arrival of British East India Company, there were reportedly no known institutions to keep the insane in India. Later their development and minimal progress reflected the interest ad perhaps neglect, by the colonialists of those days. Thus, the establishment of mental hospitals in the Indian sub-continent reflected the needs and demands of those days. It is thus believed that the institution of mental asylums in India was primarily a British concept. Accordingly, the rules and laws in respect of the admission and discharge of mental patients at that time were greatly influenced by the ideas and concepts as prevalent in England and Europe at that time.

In the early part of 20th century, there was a growing concern in the public about the conditions of mental hospitals, a desire to improve hospital conditions, and a need to open many new hospitals. Due to this awareness and the demand, the Government contemplated to have a central supervision of mental hospitals in 1906. In due course, this was brought out in the form of Indian Lunacy Act in 1912. However this legislation had a marked racial bias. Separate hospitals were established for European and Indian patients and different provisions were made for them in the law. In 1920, the names of all lunatic asylums were changed to mental hospitals and the control of mental hospitals was shifted from prison authorities to civil surgeons.

After 40 years of Independence, the Mental Health Bill, 1987 was passed by Rajya Sabha on 26th November 1986 and Lok Sabha on 19th March 1987. The amendments made by the Lok Sabha were agreed to by the Rajya Sabha on 22nd April 1987. After it was assented to on 22nd May 1987, it became Act No.14 of 1987.

Although the Act is ready for implementation only few States in the country agreed to the change and implemented the Mental Health Act of 1987, and the majority of the mental hospitals in the country even now follows only the Indian Lunacy Act of 1912.

The Indian Lunacy Act of 1912 is a legacy of the pre-scientific era and many parts of this Act need radical revisions. The details of admission into and discharge from mental hospitals found in Indian Lunacy Act of 1912 will be dealt in details in the latter part of this text (UNIT-6).

Civil responsibilities and criminal responsibilities of the mentally ill and the legal aspects of psychiatric nursing will be discussed little later. (UNIT-5).

Questions

1. Write short notes on:

   i) Exorcism

   ii) Zil Boorg

   iii) Objectives of National Mental Health Program for India.

2. Discuss the causative factors of mental illness.

3. How does Indian Lunacy Act of 1912 provided legal protection to mentally ill?

COMMUNITY RESPONSIBILITY

Attitudes towards mentally ill

The opinions and attitudes of a community towards mental illness and mentally ill carry implications for the epidemiological studies of mental disordes, as these may influence the willingness of the subjects to declare symptoms in the course of surveys of psychiatric disorders. Declaration will also depend on the prevailing concepts of mental disorders in the society and the resulting evaluation and interpretation of anomalies of behaviour.

Availability of mental health facilities do not guarantee that these services would be utilised by the population, as this is dependent on the community orientations towards mental illness. Early recognition of mental illness, enlistment of professional help at the right time, rehabilitation of the mentally ill in the community and the total involvement of the community in mental health programs' will facilitate when the attitudes, opinions held about mental illness become favourable and the attitude towards mentally ill becomes sympathetic.

The largest number of studies conducted in western countries about the attitude of public towards mentally ill reveals that there is misinformation, fear and anxiety about the mentally ill which make the public stigmatise and reject them. Mental illness is something which people want to keep away as far as possible. Community responds to mentally ill through a sequence of denial, isolation and rejection. There is also a major lack of recognition of mental illness as illness and a predominant tendency towards the rejection of both the mental patients and those who treat them.

In India, the social stigma attached to mental illness vary according to the culture.

A great deal of misconception, superstition and ignorance exists in respect of mental disease. Much stigma is often attached. Mental illnesses are viewed as a visitation of evil spirits, of a goddess, of a curse. This takes the form of exaggerated belief in mystic influences, excessive faith in the powers of saints, priests and medicaments. Among Muslims, the visitation takes the form of Sayyad. The medicaments, sorcerers, faith healers, priests, etc. are frequently engaged to cure cases of mental illness, snake bites, etc. There are a number of places of worship reputed as centres of treatment endowed with the healing power due to a deity.

Mentally ill are viewed as people with no capacity for understanding. Pessimism pervades about the possibility of a cure and if any one gets better, complete physical rest is considered essential. A sizable section in urban community rejects the mentally ill, but in the rural population there is still considerable tolerance for the mentally ill.

The general trend of the studies carried out in India so far indicates that the lay public – including the educated urban groups – are largely uninformed about the various aspects of mental health and the information possessed by them remains uncrystallised. The mentally ill are perceived as aggressive, violent and dangerous. There is a lack of desirable degree of awareness about available facilities to treat the mentally ill and a pervasive defeatism exists about the possible outcome after therapy. A tendency to maintain social distance from the mentally ill and to reject them makes its existence felt.

There are various causes of such severe rejection of patients by their families and communities.

A cause that is often adduced by the relatives themselves is economic. Looking after a chronic patient at home, even if he or she has made an appreciable degree of social recovery, is economically demanding, especially as the patient is likely to be unemployed or unemployable. But the economic reason alone is unlikely to convince anyone, considering that the same relatives would not dream of rejecting their dependent relatives, or those who are aged and infirm or who are suffering from disabling physical illnesses.

A second and an equally unconvincing reason advanced is inadequacy of living accommodation and other facilities of for day-to-day living.

The real reasons for rejection are more often unverbalised and most often, the family's rejection of a patient is actually a reflection of the rejection of the mentally ill by the society at large. Now there are many reasons for the society's large-scale rejection of the mentally ill – especially the long institutionalised mentally ill.

i) The mentally ill are deviant from the normal and therefore face the risk of rejection. In addition to being deviant from the normal, they are irrational, liable to varying degree of loss of self-control, irresponsible or poorly responsible and are often repulsive because of their bizarre behaviour.

Admission to a mental hospital tends to make the stigma associated with mental illness more ineradicable.

ii) The mentally ill patient tends to be rejected because of his substandard performance in the occupational and social spheres. In a culture where work-efficiency is an important determinant of social status, the society tends to employ the normative standards of work-performance in judging an individual's degree of social acceptability.

iii) Much of the society's rejection of the mentally ill, especially the chronic psychiatric patients, is because of the custodial type of institutional care, depriving them of all privileges, and indoctrinating them into becoming submissive, conforming, spiritless robots, without initiative or zest for living, we can scarcely expect the relatives and the society to accept them back into the community.

The stigma of hopelessness associated with psychosis in the public mind is, to be sure, sorely lamented by custodial care and its outcome leads to rejection of the mentally ill.

iv) A factor that tends to perpetuate the stigma associated with mental illness and admission to a mental hospital, in our country, at any rate is the archaic and degrading Indian Lunacy Act of 1912. The fact that inspite of efforts being put to develop The Mental Health Act, 1987, all the states have not implemented it as yet, clearly shows that even our legislators are no better than the community at large in the matter of forming better attitude towards the mentally ill.

Community responsibility

Traditional large mental hospitals may actually serve as breeding ground for secondary problems like hospitalism, in addition to continuing to serve as dumping ground for incarcerating the unwanted chronically mentally ill. Such institutions should not ever be built in future. There is enough convincing evidence to show that schizophrenic patients of all types and stages of illness can be treated successfully in smaller, open institutions situated more centrally in the community.

Home-care for psychiatric patients is feasible and the combination of drug therapy, community health nurses' home visits is effective in preventing hospitalisation. The home - care treatment model is one of the ideal models for large - scale planning in community against mental illness. Home-care has several advantageous features to offer :

35

i)   It does not disrupt the routine familial and social life of the patient.

ii) It forces the family to assume responsibility for participation in the treatment program of the patient.

iii) It enables the family to handle the problem of patient rejection in a more realistic way.

iv) The program is particularly suited to our country where the family ties have been traditionally strong and continue to be adequately preserved inspite of the adverse influence of urbanisation and industrialisation.

Development of the home-care program for large-scale use will, however, require training large numbers of para psychiatric professionals, like community health nurses trained with greater orientation toward mental health nursing and psychiatric social workers, in addition to psychiatrists.

Vocational rehabilitation of the chronically mentally ill must receive active and immediate attention of mental health professionals. The role of sheltered workshops in this connection has been well-established.

Incidentally, the community tends to underrate the performance-potentials of ex-psychiatric patients. This, combined with an over-solicitous and protective attitude tends to make us lay more emphasis on 'sheltering' rather than on the workshop element in organisation of "sheltered workshop" programs. This is actually prejudicial to the success of psychiatric rehabilitation programs. Because it was found that low-level–performance–patients tended to reside with relatives who did not expect them to work or to participate in social activities even 6 months after release from the hospital. Patients with high-performance-levels, on the other hand, tended to live with relatives who expected them to work and to be socially active within 3 months after discharge from the hospital.

Regarding the stigma associated with mental illness and mental hospitals and the rejection of the mentally ill by their relatives and society at large, there is a necessity for a mental health education program at mass level.

The emphasis has to be made that mental illness is, like physical illness, treatable by modern medical techniques and that there should be no more stigma attached to schizophrenia than, say, diabetes or appendicitis. For this, mental health professionals need to show the ex-patients as models leaving them into the community and placing them with re-employment and thorough reintegration through social skill training.

To really convince the average man of the treatability and returnability of the mentally ill patient to the community as a useful citizen, one must show concrete results. There is a need for immediate and energetic measures for rehabilitation of the more chronic patients.

To cope with the problem of rejection by the families, which is an immediate concern to us because of its intimate tie-up without discharge policy, the present policy of discharging the patient to their homes, knowing fully well that the relatives are not prepared to take their wards back, is highly prejudical to the patients' interests. We are only rendering the patients', rejection more complete thereby. It is true that our hospitals are badly over-crowded and we need the beds for more needy patients, but the answer to this problem is not in discharging the long-stay patients into the community without providing for their after-care and rehabilitation in the community. If the families won't have them back, we have to plan for their rehabilitation in an extra-familial framework.

Deploying community group homes for resettlement of unwanted ex-patient is more satisfactory than building hostels for the purpose. Group homes provide accommodation for patients who need little supervision. They are particularly suitable for chronic schizophrenics who have become independent of the hospital but cannot live on their own or with their families. Group homes are ordinary houses in residential areas. Five or six patients live together, sharing domestic tasks according to their abilities. Community nurses visit regularly, but as much responsibility as possible is left to the residents. Success depends on discrete supervision and careful selection of patients who are to live closely together.

Whereas the hostels built for chronic patients may give rise to further isolation of patients from community for the following reasons :

i) The hostels, though they may be situated in the heart of the community, are likely to be looked upon as refined "miniature hospitals" because of isolation of the residents in one building and cutting them off from the stream of community living. This is only likely to perpetuate the stigma associated with mental illness.

ii) The resident is likely to take longer to gain confidence in social competence, because of the less demanding atmosphere in a hostel.

iii) Deploying a boarding house is more effective and quicker way of minimising the community's rejection of the mentally ill and also of ensuring the community's participation in the community-based treatment program for the mentally ill.

iv) Boarding-house/group homes method of resettlement is economically more advantageous.

Hostels, however, do have a place in the resettlement programs for the chronically ill, especially as half-way houses for certain patients who can't make the grade to boarding houses straight from hospital, or for those patients who are too ill to stay in boarding houses but at the same time not ill enough to continue to stay in hospital.

Re-socialisation of mentally ill patients do not need much technical expertise an it is actually advantageous to have non-professional people from the community like volunteers, community leaders etc., as they are likely to be more spontaneous and on this account, the patients will be exposed to variegated types of individual personalities and this will make their subsequent re-entry into community and social functioning easier.

Employing volunteers for services of the mentally ill is also a method of over-coming the community's resistance to the mentally ill and ensuring a greater community participation in the treatment programs for the chronically ill.

Our community attitude towards mentally ill is gradually changing. A greater degree of commitment on the part of mental health professionals including nurses in the matter of rehabilitation measures for the chronic patients and providing dynamic therapeutic communities, and making the community to become self-reliant would further change the attitude of community towards mental illness in a more acceptable manner.

Misconceptions towards mentally ill

When our attitudes towards understanding and accepting mental illness are examined over centuries, we find that they have not progressed dramatically. Our approaches to the mentally ill are determined not only by medical and psychiatric theories, but also by the legislation and social climate of the time.

In recent years court decisions have affirmed individual's right to treatment, right to refuse treatment and right to treatment in the least restrictive setting. These rulings influence our attitudes about mentally disturbed persons and their rights and responsibilities.

An individual's values and personal beliefs affect his attitudes about mental illness, people with mental disorders and treatment of mental illness. There still exists a stigma surrounding individuals who need or use psychiatric mental health services. The need continues for public education to modify or alter misconceptions about mental illness and persons with mental disorders.

Beliefs about mental illness have been characterised by superstitions, ignorance and fear. Although time and again advances in scientific understanding of mental illness have dispelled many false ideas, there remain a number of popular misconceptions, and they are :

i) Mentally ill people show bizarre behaviour

Patients in mental hospitals and clinics are often picturised as a weird lot who spent their time doing useless bizarre behaviour like twisting the hands, passing one hand fingers to another hand fingers and folding the hands together at the back etc.

ii) Mentally ill people are unstable and dangerous

This goes along with another false belief that mental disorders are incurable. So people who have had a mental illness are viewed with suspicion and as dangerous persons.

iii) Mental illness is something to be ashamed

This idea arouses a unsympathetic, cruel attitude towards a mentally ill person. This is the reason why many people hide the mental illness in the family.

iv) Mental illness is caused by supernatural power forces provoked or unprovoked by patients, or it is a result of curse or possession of evil spirits

Many people consider that mental illness is not an illness but possession by spirit, or dead. They also believe that a person becomes mentally ill, because he broke a taboo. Still another notion is that mental illness is caused by curse that is befallen on the patient or family for the past sin or misdeed of previous life.

v) Mental illness is something that cannot be cured and it is contagious

Not only is the person looked at with suspicion, but people object to have normal relations with mentally ill, to give him employment even after cured or even to accept him as a neighbour. The fear that it is contagious

41

is the main false notion which leads the family members also being eyed suspiciously or object marital relations with a person belong to the household of the mentally ill. (eg. daughter) and where the family is looked down and obstracised.

vi) An exaggerated fear of one's own susceptibility to oriental disorder

Fear of possible mental disorder is very common cause which leads to needless unhappiness, anxiety and which causes alarm in people.

vii) Mental illness are caused by evil spirits, black magic, witchcraft, influence of bad stars and bad deeds committed in the past or present life

Therefore, they seek the help of faith healers, mantravadis and magicians who perform pujas, counter-magic, exorcism, offer prayers to Gods or give native/herbal medicines.

Most people do not make use of even the available limited facilities for treating mental illness. It is estimated that less than 10 per cent of patients who need help, actually take modern treatment. A large majority of patients remain without getting help of any sort because of ignorance, fear, stigma, misconceptions or wrong beliefs regarding the causes and treatment of mental illness.

viii) Mental hospitals are places where only dangerous mentally ill individuals are treated with restraint as a major approach

People have fear about mental hospitals. Hence they hesitate to take their relatives to these hospitals for treatment. Further an ex-patient of a mental hospital as well

42

as his family members are often socially isolated and stigmatised. Therefore, people seek help from mental hospitals only as a last resort.

ix) Mental illness is hereditary

Children of mentally ill persons do not necessarily become mentally ill. Children of most patients remain healthy and lead a normal life.

x) Marriage can cure mental illness

A mentally ill person can get worse if he gets married when he is ill. Marriage can become an additional stress. A patient who has recovered can get married and live a normal life like any other person.

All the misconception regarding mental illness has brought a social 'stigma' to this illness. And thus, the attitude of people towards mental illness is always one that is associated with negative community reactions, such as harsh, cruel, unsympathetic, indifferent reactions which leads to 'hiding of the illness' or 'resisting the patient' and treating him secretly through non-medico professional means and there is social rejection of the patient in the family.

Health and social services for the mentally sick

India is a signatory state to the Alma Ata Declaration which envisaged health for all by the year 2000 A.D. as the goal. Efforts to ensure the achievement of this goal will have to include approaches and strategies for the improvement of all aspects of health–physical, mental and social. While the Government of

India is fully seized with the formulation of a national health policy and mental health forms an integral part of total health, a plan of action aiming at the mental health component of the national health program, needs to be put forward.

The importance of mental health cannot be over-emphasised in the national health planning. The scope of mental health is not only confined to the treatment of some seriously mentally ill persons admitted to mental hospitals but it also relates to the whole range of health activities.

Following major scientific discoveries in the field of psychotropic drugs, physical methods of treatment, psychotherapy and other behaviour modification techniques, simple, effective and cheap methods of treatment are now available for a large number of serious and disabling mental disorders.

Existing Mental Health Services

i)   Hospital

The presently available mental health facilities in India include about 20,000 beds in 42 mental hospitals and 2000 to 3000 psychiatric beds in general and teaching hospitals. For an estimated population 860 million, there is one psychiatric bed per 32,500 population.

ii)   Community

Mental health services in a community are concerned not only with early diagnosis and treatment, but also with the preservation and promotion of good mental health and prevention of mental illness.

Since 95 per cent of psychiatric cases can be treated with or without hospitalisation close to their homes, the current trend is full integration of psychiatric services with other health services. The community mental health program includes all community facilities pertinent in any way to prevention, treatment and rehabilitation.

iii) In-patient psychiatric care

It is currently undergoing major changes. The hospital has become a part of a continuum of mental health services available to patients and their families. It offers a variety of therapies in the treatment of psychiatric and behavioural disorders. To name a few,

a) **Milieu therapy** is a "scientific manipula tion of the environment aimed at produc ing changes in the personality of the pa tient". The word "milieu" was first used to mean a scientifically planned environment by Bettlcheim and Sylvester in the late 1930's and early 1940's.

b) **Therapeutic community** is a "very special kind of milieu therapy in which the total social structure of the treatment unit is involved as part of the helping process". In this, all social and interpersonal inter-actions in the hospital are the main thera-peutic tools used to bring about specific changes in the patient.

Characteristics of a therapeutic environ ment are that it : (1) encourages a client to participate in his/her own plan of care, (2) helps the client gain new insights about

45

self, (3) allows the client to test new patterns of behaviour, (4) is accepting, (5) is democratic, and (6) provides adequate protection.

Elements of a therapeutic milieu include open communication between clients and staff and among staff, individualisation of treatment programs, and often some form of ward government led by clients. The self-government system implies that the clients will have some degree of input into planning daily activities, setting policies, orienting newly admitted clients, and in some cases making decisions about fellow patients, such as appropriateness of week end pass or time of discharge.

c) **Family therapy** : The focus of family therapy is to treat a social system as the primary unit, rather than an individual member who has been defined as a "patient".

The goals of family therapy are to reduce conflict and anxiety, to make the family members more aware of each other's needs, to increase the family's ability to deal with external and internal crises, to develop more appropriate role relationships, to help individual family members cope with destructive forces within and outside the family, and to promote health and growth.

d) **Psychotherapy** : There are various types of psychotherapy based on various aim, purpose and intensity. Mainly individual psychotherapy and group psychotherapy are conducted. They are given to reconstruct the personality of patients.

e) **Rehabilitation therapies** : A number of vital programs fall under the general classification of rehabilitation therapies. These programs are used on an active in-patient psychiatric unit as either adjunctive or primary treatment modalities.

Adjunctive therapies mainly are,

A. **Occupational therapy** : It is defined as the art and science of directing a person's participation in selected activity to diminish or correct pathological problems and promote and maintain health.

B. **Recreational therapy** : It is usually geared towards physical or gamelike activities. The theory holds that the relationship of one's physical self to the immediate environment is important to the individual's total health. Organised tournaments in volley ball, basket ball, table tennis, cards, etc. provide the patients with useful leisure activities and help them develop skills in engaging in healthy, competitive interactions.

C. **Art therapy** is used as both a diagnostic tool and a treatment modality. The art therapist's goals are to help the patient express his thoughts and emotions through his drawings, to help the patient gain relief from anxiety by graphically representing conflicts and aggressive, and traumatic material without guilt, to provide a socially acceptable outlet for fantasy and wish fulfillment, and to help the patient develop more dexterity.

D. **Pet and Horticultural therapy** is to allow the patient to express tender, loving and nurturing feelings without great fear of rejection. Plants and pets respond well to care but make fewer demands than families and friends. Through this form of therapy patients become alerted to the needs of other living organisms and may develop a sensitivity and sense of responsibility to respond to these needs in an appropriate manner.

E. **Poetry therapy** is the use of poetry in a group setting, both writing it and reading it, to enable clients to work together and to gain insights into their behaviour. Poetry may help the client get in touch with feelings through expression or through seeing parallels in the writings of others.

F. **Music therapy** offers the challenge of expansion of knowledge; provides the discipline of orderly activity; promotes improvement in concentration, attention span, and memory; and provides pride of achievement.

G. **Dance therapy** is the psychotherapeutic use of movement as a process which enhances emotional and physical integration of the individual. The focus is on developing individual body awareness, group inter-action and co-operation and sharing of feelings in movement.

H. **Bibliotherapy** : In this, the patient is assisted to broaden experiences, see parallels with personal life, and perhaps assimilate values from books into his/her own life, in addition to providing a medium for discussions with others.

All of these rehabilitation therapies help patients develop occupational and leisure skills that provide a smoother transition back into the community. They also provide non-threatening media to the patient and provide the opportunity to decrease inhibitions, share values at a feeling level, and allow vicarious experience of a variety of life experiences.

J. Somatic therapies and psycho pharmacology : Chemotherapy and Electro-convulsive therapy (ECT) are the most frequently used of all the somatic treatments.

iv) Partial hospitalisation

It is another treatment alternative. It has an advantage of less separation from families, more family involvement in the treatment program, and a lessening of the patient's preoccupation with the illness, which may be intensified by full hospitalisation.

Day hospital, Evening hospital and Night hospital are few examples for partial hospitalisation.

The week-end care center is another form of partial hospitalisation wherein patients may devote week days to their usual pursuits and obtain intensive treatment on Saturday and Sunday. This program is particularly useful for patients who do not require in-patient care but who live too far from a treatment centre to obtain day care.

v) Community homes

There are small, home like residential centres where groups of recovered patients stay together and maintain their daily livings. It offers strict to minimum protection, depending on the needs of the residents.

vi) Half way homes

They offer a variety of therapies, facilities, transition between the hospital and independent living where the person is without the benefit of therapy except for weekly counseling sessions or maintenance drug therapy.

Problems that discharged patients from hospital have when they live in the community residential facilities are (a) reduced social competence, (b) alienation from significant others, (c) loss of supportive systems in society due to their absence from society, and (d) extrusion or rejection by the community.

Social services for the mentally sick must assist for establishing social linkability. It is an act of joining a human being with other human beings, agencies, or community resources with the aim of reintegrating and maintaining him/her in the society or community.

Social linkability is to give to a former mental hospital patient, a sense of belonging and involvement, and a means of satisfying the need for respect, identity, and status.

Questions

1. Discuss in brief the general attitude of community towards mentally ill.

2. Enumerate the reasons for the society's large-scale rejection of mentally ill.

3. Outline the mental health services that are available in the community for rehabilitating mentally ill.

4. List down the misconceptions towards mentally ill.

5. What are the mental health services available for the in-patients in the hospital?

6. Write short notes on :

   i) Community homes

   ii) Half way homes

   iii) Therapeutic community.

UNIT 4

DIAGNOSIS

Early recognition of deviations from the normal

Psychiatric nursing is a branch of nursing that deals with the care of psychiatric patients who are considered as abnormal in their behaviour. Abnormality is a negative concept. Terms like "Psychopathology", "maladaptive behaviour", "disordered behaviour", "deviancy", etc. can all be equated with term "abnormal".

Abnormal means "deviation" or different from the "norm" or "standard". So the abnormal behaviour could be explained within the framework of the normal and the general. To conceptualise abnormal behaviour few major models like medical model, statistical model and socio-cultural model are used.

The term "normal" is derived from the Latin word "Norma", which refers to a carpenter's square or rule. It implies deviation from `norm' or `standard' as abnormal.

Defining the concepts of 'normal' and abnormal behaviour is found to be difficult. Whereas it appears to be possible to define in hard science like physics or chemistry. For example, in the nursing practice, when a temperature of patient is 37° celsius, we call it as normal and wide deviations such as 35° C or 40° C, would be considered as abnormal needing immediate medical attention. Such standard measurement is universal. But there are areas where these concepts are influenced by socio-cultural factors. For instance, in Indian hospitals, it is common to see most of the people weiling at their chest and crying for the death of a significant person in the family. They are however considered to be normal by us. But the same behaviour is considered to be abnormal by Americans. Similarly, there are several dimensions related to distinguish the concepts of abnormal from normal.

In general

All of us get emotionally disturbed at different times due to a variety of reasons. Sometimes we feel sad while at other times, we experience tension and anxiety. We get irritable, angry and occasionally behave peculiarly in response to certain situations. Usually, such behaviours do not disturb others. These day to day changes are not considered to be abnormal. Such reactions are considered as being "off mood", "emotional upset", "losing temper", etc.

Generally behaviour is considered abnormal and is suggestive of mental illness when it occurs without an understandable reason, it is exaggerated, it lasts for a long time and causes disability to the individual or others.

There are few characteristics which help us to recognise deviations from normal. They are,

(i)   Recurrent changes in one's thinking, feel ing, memory, perceptions and judgement resulting in abnormalities in talk and behaviour.

(ii) Those changes cause distress and suffering to the individual or others around him or both.

(iii) The changed behaviour and the consequent distress cause disturbances in day to day activities, work efficiency, and relationship with others (social and occupational disability).

For example, most students become anxious at the time of examinations. They are worried whether they would pass and are afraid of the consequences of failure. Yet majority of them them take the examination. Only a few become so anxious that they cannot study. Such students complain that they forget whatever they read and often stay away from the examination. They are unable to sleep soundly. They become increasingly worried about their difficulties. The later group can be considered to have an emotional illness.

It is natural for a mother to feel sad when a child or close family member dies. She may not eat properly or sleep well and can be disinterested in routine life. This may continue for about 3 to 4 weeks, after which she gradually accepts the loss and starts attending to her daily work once again. But if she continues to feel sad about the death, frequently weeps, neglects the other children and the household work for many months after the loss, her sadness is considered "abnormal" and a feature of mental illness.

Occasionally, individuals may be unable to sleep or fail to eat properly due to poor appetite. By straining themselves or thinking too much some persons get a headache and feel exhausted. These experiences usually last only for short periods of time. But if they recur frequently and last for long periods of time, they can become disturbing. They could then be considered as a "feature of mental illness". Therefore, for a person to be considered mentally ill, he should have symptoms which bother him and/or other around him and disturb his daily routines.

Conceptual models

They are organisation of complex body of knowledge. No model is said to be superior to other as no scientific study proved so far. And also abnormal behaviour is based on social norms and the self expectation of an individual. Thereby behaviour is defined as normal or abnormal in terms of the degree of deviation and not in terms of its kind.

Medical model

Medical model considers organic pathology as the definite cause for the mental disorder. All persons suffering from mental disorder are considered to be abnormal, unhealthy and ineffective. This concept of mental illness is called the organic view point or medical model. Abnormal people are the ones who have disturbances in thought, conation, perceptions and psycho motor activities. The normal are the ones free from these disturbances.

The medical model· has been very useful in simplifying treatment practices and in contributing to improved methods of controlling diseases – both physical and mental.

Pathological symptoms vary in degrees from individual to individual. Hence at what degree he or she has to be told as abnormal is not explained in this model.

The pathophysiological explanation of organic psychosis could be considered relevant to explain the deviations in normal behaviour. Any change either in the structure or functions of the brain can cause mental illness. Biochemical changes at the level of the nerve cells are the cause in a majority of the severe type of mental illnesses (Psychosis).

As we have earlier discussed any damage to the brain due to any of the following reasons can also cause mental illness: (a) infections (b) injury (c) poor blood supply (d) bleeding (e) tumours (f) alcohol intake for long periods (g) vitamin deficiencies, and (h) untreated epilepsy.

Statistical model

It involves the analyses of responses on a test or a questionnaire or observations on some particular behavioural variable or variables. The degree of deviation from the standard norms, arrived at statistically, characterises the degree of abnormality. For example, in the case of intelligence, where an intelligent quotient (IQ) of 100 is considered as normal, interpreting the measures at the two ends of the normal distribution curve becomes difficult. (See the figure below). An IQ of 150, which is above average, becomes an index of abnormality when the statistical criterion is applied to it.

Low IQ may be a proper subject for study by clinical psychologist, but can the opposite, high IQ be considered as abnormal?

Hence this model also has the draw back that when the statistical model is adopted the question of

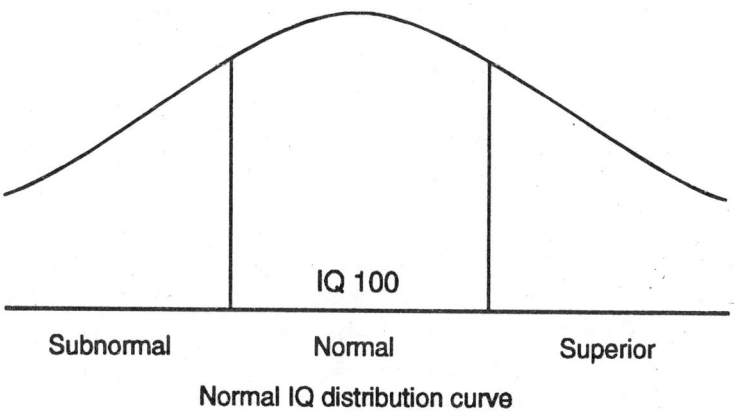

IQ 100

Subnormal   Normal   Superior

Normal IQ distribution curve

establishing point beyond which behaviour is regarded as abnormal must also be considered. Therefore, although providing a partial description of abnormality, the statistical model must be considered rather inadequate.

In some mental illnesses, intelligence and the ability to take decisions deteriorate. Patient loses his reasoning skills and abilities. He makes mistakes in his routine work. He is not able to do simple arithmetic and reacts like a dull person.

Among the psychiatric illnesses, mental retardation is considered as a subnormal state of intelligence. It is not an illness but a condition of poor development of the brain. Children who have this condition are called dull or mentally retarded. Therefore statistical model is being used to recognise the deviation of persons from normal.

Socio-cultural model

The beliefs, norms, taboos and values of a society have to be accepted and adopted by individuals. Breaking any of these would be considered as abnormal. For example, humbleness is normal among Hindus but would be considered as abnormal in the aggressive and competitive climate of the west. So normalcy is defined in context with social norms prescribed by the culture. Thus cultural background has to be taken into account in distinguishing between the normal and abnormal behaviour.

Every individual behaves in a given situation based upon his physical competencies and the type of learning he has from the society. Only when he fails to adjust to himself or/and with others in the society, he is said to be abnormal or mentally ill.

There are marked features to indicate individual's deviations from the normal in the area of physiological function, mental function and one's attitude towards himself and in relation to social activities.

(i) **Features of disturbances in bodily functions**

    a)   **Sleep :** The patient finds it difficult to get sleep. He lies on the bed or sits and worries for not getting sleep. He wakes up in the middle of the night and fails to get sleep again. He has disturbed sleep throughout the night or he does not sleep at all. He is not fresh in the morning. Any of these types of sleep disturbances can be present.

b) **Appetite and food intake** : Patient does not have appetite and eats less, or although he has appetite he does not relish what he eats. He loses weight too.

c) **Bowel and bladder movements** : Patient passes urine more frequently than before. He has loose motions or becomes constipated. Some patients soil their clothes. They re main unaware of it.

d) **Sexual desire and activity** : Patient loses interest in sex. He can become impotent too.

(ii) Changes in mental functions

Patients have disturbance of irrelevant talk, excessively sad or happy, abnormal perception of hearing or seeing, etc. They appear to be unaware of everything and be talking or laughing to self. This indicates that the person is suffering from mental illness.

(iii) Changes in individual and social activities

Patient neglects his personal needs regular bath, food intake and stays mute and asocial. Some other patients may hurt others including family members with their hyper activities and do not conduct themselves in a socially approved manner.

The observations of these kind become helpful for early recognition of deviation from normal.

Classification of mental disorders

In the early 1960's the Mental Health Program of the World Health Organisation (WHO) became actively engaged in a programme, improve the diagnosis and classification of mental disorders. Numerous proposals to improve the classification of mental disorders resulted from the extensive consultation process and these were used in drafting the Eighth Revision of the International Classification of Diseases (ICD-8).

The 1970's saw further growth of interest in improving psychiatric classification world wide. In 1979, WHO again brought out another classification called ICD-9. Most of the psychiatric hospital use this ICD-9 currently for diagnosis of patients with mental disorder. In 1987, further refinement brought out ICD-10, chapter V (F) and that is being used in a few hospitals.

ICD-10 is much larger than ICD-9. Numeric codes (001-999) were used in ICD-9, whereas an alpha numeric coding scheme, based on codes with a single letter followed by two numbers at the three-character level (A00-Z99), has been adopted in ICD-10. This has significantly enlarged the number of categories available for the classification. The chapter on mental disorders in ICD-9 had only 30 three-character categories (290-319); whereas chapter V (F) of ICD-10 has 100 such categories with decimal numeric subdivisions at the four-character level.

ICD-10 gives the description of the main clinical features, diagnostic guidelines and clinical description.

The main categories in the draft of ICD-10 are as follows :

F00 - F09 Organic, including symptomatic, mental disorders

Dementia

Delirium

Amnestic syndrome

F10 - F19 Mental and behavioural disorders due to psycho active substance use

Alcohol and drug use

F20 - F29 Schizophrenia, Schizotypal and delusional disorders

Schizophrenia

Schizotypal disorder

Persistent delusional disorders

Acute and transient psychotic disorders.

F30 - F39 Mood (Affective) disorders

Manic episode

Pripolar affective disorder

Depressive episode

Recurrent depressive disorder

Persistent mood (affective) disorders

F40 - F48 Neurotic, stress-related and somato form disorders

Phobic anxiety disorders

Other anxiety disorders

Obsessive-compulsive disorder

Reaction to severe stress, and adjustment disorders

Dissociative (conversion) disorders

Somatoform disorders

Other neurotic disorders.

F50 - F59 Behavioural syndromes associated with physiological disturbances and physical factors.

Eating disorders

Non organic sleep disorders

Sexual dysfunction, not caused by organic disorder or disease.

Mental and behavioural disorders associated with the puerperium not elsewhere classified.

F60 - F69 Disorders of adult personality and behaviour

Specific personality disorders

Mixed and other personality disorders

Enduring personality changes not attributable to brain damage and disease

Habit and impulse disorders

Gender identity disorders

Disorders of sexual preference

F70 - F79 Mental retardation

Mild mental retardation

Moderate mental retardation

Severe mental retardation

Profound mental retardation

F80 - F89 Disorders of psychological development

Specific developmental disorders of speech and language

Specific developmental disorders of scholastic skills

Specific developmental disorders of motor function

Mixed specific developmental disorders

Pervasive developmental disorders

F90 – F98 Behavioural and emotional disorders with onset usually occurring in childhood and adolescence

Hyperkinetic disorders

Conduct disorders

Mixed disorders of conduct and emotions

Emotional disorders with onset specific to childhood

Disorders of social functioning with onset specific to childhood and adolescence

Tic disorders

Other behavioural and emotional disorders with onset usually occurring in childhood and adolescence.

F99 Unspecified mental disorder

Diagnostic and Statistical Manual (DSM)

The American Psychiatric Association had also contributed to the classification of mental diseases. It brought out its revised DSM-II in 1968. This classification was based on the comparisons of the incidence, types of disorders and treatment procedures. It identifies the premorbid personality, external stress and the degree of impairment. Attempts at further revision of this classification have resulted in the emergence of DSM-III (1980). With remedy to some of the faults of DSM-III, DSM-IIIR has been produced.

Indian classification

In India Neki (1963), Wig and Singer (1967), Vahia (1961) and Varma (1971) have attempted some modifications of ICD-8 to suit Indian conditions. They are broadly grouped as follows: (See figure on page 66).

i) Psychosis

— Functional —— Simple schizophrenia,
Hebephrenic schizophrenia,
Catatonic schizophrenia,
paranoid schizophrenia

—— Affective

Mania   Depression - Unipolar,
Bipolar and Cyclic

—— Organic ——— Acute and chronic

ii) Neurosis

- Anxiety neurosis
- Depressive neurosis
- Hysterical neurosis
- Obsessive-compulsive neurosis
- Phobic neurosis.

iii) Special disorders like

a) Childhood disorders – conduct & emotional disorders.

b) Personality disorders – sociopath & psychopath.

c) Substance abuses – Alcohol and drugs

d) Psycho physiological disorders – Asthma, psoriasis.

e) Mental retardation – Mild, moderate, severe & profound

To remove the difficulties in communication due to different classification in different countries, WHO brought out ICD.

In every day practice, classification is made after the history and examination of mental state have been completed. The first step is to review the pattern of the symptoms occurring in the past month (as reported by the patient and any other informants) and of the symptoms and signs elicited by mental state examination. Then an attempt is made to match this pattern to one or more of the diagnostic categories in the system of the classification used. In practice, only a small number of categories need be considered, the rest being obviously inapplicable.

Classification of Mental Illness

Psychosis	Neurosis	Special Disorders
Functional Organic	Anxiety neurosis	Childhood disorders
Affective	Depressive neurosis	(Conduct & emotional)
Mania Depression Acute Chronic	Hysterical neurosis	Personality disorders
(Unipolar, Bipolar & Cyclic)	Obsessive compulsive neurosis	(Sociopath, Psychopath)
Schizophrenia	Phobic neurosis	Substance abuses
Simple Hebephrenic Catatonic Paranoid		(Alcohol, drugs)
		Psychopsysiological disorders
		(Asthma, psoriasis)
		Mental retardation
		(Mild, moderate, severe, profound)

Psychosis

It is a severe type of mental illness in which the patient talks and behaves abnormally. The functions of the body and mind are severely disturbed resulting in gross impairment of individual and social activities. He loses touch with reality and people label him as 'mad'. He is not aware of his illness and can refuse to take treatment.

Psychosis is further divided into :

i) **Functional psychosis** (eg. schizophrenia)

Schizophrenia is the commonest of the psychoses and its symptoms closely correspond to the layman's concept of mental illness. It is an illness which interferes with the individual's personal and social functioning and if untreated, runs a chronic course. The illness is characterised by abnormalities of thinking, perceptions and emotions resulting in abnormal behaviour, action and talk. The schizophrenic has abnormal ideas and thoughts of various kinds which he firmly believes in and are unshakable (delusions). He perceives things which really do not exist (that is he hears voices and sees visions which are not existent – auditory hallucination and visual hallucination, respectively). He misinterprets the environment and has special meanings for various things of normal occurance. He may be unusually happy or sad inappropriately a apathetic and unconcerned. Because of these, his talk and actions might become ununderstandable and irrelevant. He may either talk too much (pressure of speech) or too little or not talk at all (mute). He may be found talking and laughing to self. This can be his responding to the voices he hears. He may be withdrawn and inactive or restless and hyperactive. (Disturbances in psycho motor

67

activities). He may become suddenly hostile, abusive and assaultive in response to an unpleasant thought or voice. Phases of excitement may be followed by phases of extreme withdrawal when patient may remain in uncomfortable and bizarre postures for long periods of time. Varying degrees of sleep disturbance will always be present.

It is very essential to remember that in actual clinical practice, only some of the above features may be present in any given patient.

ii) Affective psychosis

Affective psychosis is named to a condition where the primary abnormality in the illness is one of 'affect' (affect = emotion, mood). Manic depressive psychosis is the main condition seen in affective psychosis. The disturbance in mood occurs both of quality and quantity and ranges from extreme sadness to extreme happiness. The mood disturbance occurs in episodes of either happiness (mania) or sadness (depression). These episodes can also occur alternatingly when the illness is called manic depressive psychosis (MDP). In between the episodes the person remains absolutely normal. A person may get only attacks of mania or only attacks of depression (unipolar) or both alternatingly (bipolar). By and large recurrent attacks of depression is the commonest manifestation of affective illness (cyclic) and only a quarter of all affective psychoses occur classically as alternating attacks of mania and depression (MDP).

iii) Organic psychosis

These are otherwise known as 'organic brain disorder'. They may be classified as 'acute' and 'chronic' based on the brain pathology.

Acute brain disorders are caused by diffused impairment of brain function which may result from variety of conditions such as drug intoxication, nutritional deficiencies, mild head injury, etc.

Chronic brain disorders involve permanent destruction of brain tissue as a result of brain injury, degenerative disease of the central nervous system (such as senile dementia, Parkinson's disease, etc.) intra cranial space occupying lesions, drug intoxication, etc.

Neurosis

Neuroses are a group of minor mental disorders, which are not easily defined. Unlike in psychoses, persons suffering from neuroses do not lose touch with reality and they are able to meet the ordinary demands of every day living. Neurotic people do not cause much touble to others (in the family, neighbourhood etc.) but they themselves experience varying degrees of personal distress and suffering.

The common form of neuroses are as follows:

i)   Anxiety neurosis

The predominant feature in this neurosis is a constant feeling of uneasiness, tension and apprehension with anxious anticipation of danger (when there is no real threat or danger). This anxiety state is often associated with various symptoms like tightness and beating in the chest, empty feeling in the stomach, shortness of breath, inability to concentrate, forgetfulness, disturbed sleep, nightmare, poor appetite, giddiness, weakness, excessive sweating, sustained muscle tension causing aches and pains, chronic mild diarrhoea and difficulty in making decisions. These symptoms sometimes appear in episodes and then it is known as acute anxiety or panic attack.

ii) Depressive neurosis

The commonest feature in depressive neurosis is one of sadness (depression) and worry of varying intensity. Environmental factors causing prolonged stress and strain leading to depression are invariably present. These may be family quarrels, serious illnesses or death in the family (or to close friends) financial difficulties or difficulties at work.

Usually patient complaints of lethargy, weakness, helplessness, hopelessness, decreased or lack of interest in work, people and everything around, lack of confidence, irritability, multiple bodily complaints, disturbances in sleep and lack of appetite. When the degree of sadness increases, patient may make suicidal attempts.

iii) Hysterical neurosis

Hysterical patients develop typical symptoms of physical illnesses without any evidence of any organic pathology. The illness usually helps the individual to escape or avoid a threatening or stressful situation. The stress or threat need not always be external. It may, arise from the individual's inner conflicts, impulses and desires. The symptoms, in addition to avoiding stress, may also help the individual to fulfill certain needs. They help him to draw the attention of significant members in the family and community and gain their sympathies and support. Thus, hysterical symptoms may be considered as a way of communicating distress, expressing problems or recording protests.

Hysterical symptoms can mimic any known physical illness but detailed examination would never reveal any signs of the illnesses. Management involves removal of the hysterical symptoms with suggestion and psychological support. Very often, more than the patient, it is the relatives who are concerned and who need to be reassured.

iv) Obsessive-compulsive neurosis (OCN)

In this, patient gets persistent thoughts or impulses which he himself recognises as irrational. The persistant thoughts are compelling him to indulge in meaningless activities like repeated hand washing, plates cleaning, etc.

These obsessional thoughts or ideas, images or impulses that enter the individual's mind again and again in a stereotyped form. They are almost invariably distressing and he tries to resist them. Compulsive acts or rituals are stereotyped behaviours that are repeated again and again. They are not inherently enjoyable, nor do they result in the completion of inherently useful tasks. Individuals with OCN often have depressive symptoms and patients suffering from recurrent depressive disorder may develop obsessional thoughts during their episodes of depression.

v) Phobic neurosis

The patients with phobic neurosis develop intense irrational fear of a specific object or situation, that normally presents no real danger and actively avoids the object or situation. Patients know that their fear is absolutely silly and there are no reason for fear, but still they cannot help avoiding the object or situation. Symptoms and signs of acute anxiety appear, if they ever attempt to approach the feared object or situation. For example, the patient can have phobia towards pet animals like cat or dog.

The features of anxiety may vary in severity from mild unease to terror. The individual's concern may focus on individual symptoms such as palpitations or feeling faint, and is often associated with secondary fears of dying, losing control or going mad.

Special disorders

i) Childhood disorders

Children can also have mental illness which is manifested in the form of behavioural problems like overactiveness, bed wetting, antisocial activities, scholastic backwardness, etc.

ii) Personality disorders

They are a group of disorders characterised by deeply ingrained, socially maladaptive behaviours, generally recognisable by the time of adolescence or earlier and continuing throughout or most of adult life. This category of disorders include antisocial personality, alcoholism, drug dependence and sexual deviations.

Antisocial personality people are mostly ego-centric, impulsive, irresponsible, prone to thrill seeking, poor in judgement, devoid of anxiety or guilt, unable to learn from mistake, hostile towards authority and a great burden on the family.

iii) Substance abuse

It refers to behavioural changes associated with more or less regular use of substances that effect the central nervous system. As a consequence of substance abuse, the patient has impairment in social or occupational functions and inability to control the use of or the stop taking the substance. There is a development of serious withdrawal symptoms after cessation of or reduction in substance use.

iv) Psycho physiological disorders

The main feature of this is repeated presentation of physical symptoms by patients as if they were due to a physical disorder of a system or organ that is largely or completely under autonomic innervation and control, i.e., the cardiovascular, gastro-intestinal or respiratory system.

The most common and striking examples affect the cardiovascular system ("cardiac neurosis"), the respiratory system (psychogenic hyperventilation and hiccough) and the gastro-intestinal system ("gastric neurosis" and "nervous diarrhoea").

In many patients with this disorder there will also be evidence of psychological stress, or current difficulties and problems that appear to be related to the disorder. In some of these disorders, minor disturbance of physiological function may also be present, such as hiccough, flatulence and hyperventilation, but these do not of themselves disturb the essential physiological function of the relevant organ or system.

v) Mental retardation

It is a subnormal state of intelligence. It is a condition and not a disease. There is a poor development of the brain. Mental retardation is characterised by impairment of skills manifested during the developmental period, which contribute to the overall level of intelligence, i.e., cognitive, language, motor and social activities. Retardation can occur with or without any other mental or physical disorder. Adaptive behaviour is always impaired, but in protected social environments where support is available this impairment may not be at all obvious in subjects with mild mental retardation.

Signs and symptoms of common mental illnesses

The nurse can acquire skill in examining the patients only if she has a sound knowledge of signs and symptoms of illnesses. She should determine whether the clinical features form a syndrome, which is a group of symptoms and signs that identifies patients with the specific mental illness.

Symptoms are often recognised as indicating mental illness because of their intensity and persistence. Nonetheless, even when intense and persistent, a single symptom does not necessarily indicate illness. It is the characteristic grouping of symptoms into a syndrome that is important.

A. Disorders of perception

The most distinctive phenomenon in mental illness are disorders of perception. They are,

i) **Illusions** : Illusions are misperceptions of external stimuli. They are most likely to occur when the general level of sensory stimulation is reduced or when the level of consciousness is reduced as, for example, in an acute organic syndrome. A delirious patient may mistake inanimate objects for people when the level of illumination is normal, though he is more likely to do so if the room is badly lit. Illusions occur more often when attention is not focused on the sensory modality or when there is a strong affective state (affect illusions). For example, in a dark lane a frightened person is more likely to misperceive the outline of a bush as that of an attacker.

ii) **Hallucinations** : A hallucination is a percept experienced in the absence of an external stimulus to the sense organs. Hallucinations may depend on the type of sensory system affected e.g. auditory, visual, olfactory, gustatory, tactile.

Auditory hallucinations may be experienced as noises, music or voices. Voices may be heard clearly or indistincty; they may seem to speak words, phrases or sentences; and they may seem to address the patient or talk to one another referring to the patient as 'he' or 'she'. It is common in Schizophrenia.

Visual hallucinations : It may be experienced as seeing persons, objects or animals. They may appear to be normal or abnormal size. Visual hallucinations may occur in severe affective disorders and schizophrenia, but they should always raise the possibility of an organic disorder.

Olfactory hallucinations are frequently experienced as unpleasant smells, while **Gustatory hallucinations** may be experienced with unpleasant tastes.

Hallucinations of taste and smell are infrequent. When they do occur, they often have an unusual quality which patients have difficulty in describing. They may occur in schizophrenia or severe depressive disorders, but they should also suggest temporal lobe epilepsy or irritation of the olfactory bulb or pathways by a tumour.

Tactile hallucinations may be experienced as sensations of being touched, pricked or strangled. They may also be felt as movements just below the skin which the patient may attribute to insects, worms or other small creatures burrowing through tissues. Hallucinations of deep sensation may occur as feelings of the viscera being pulled upon or distended or of sexual stimulation or electric shocks.

The sensation of insects moving under the skin occurs in people who abuse cocaine and occasionally among schizophrenics.

B. Disorders of thinking

Disorders of thinking are usually recognised from speech and writing. The term disorder of thinking can be used in a wide sense to denote four separate groups of phenomena. They are as follows :

i)   The first group comprises particular kinds of abnormal thinking – delusions and obsessional thoughts.

ii)   The second group, disorders of the stream of thought, is concerned with abnormalities of the amount and the speed of the thought experienced (speed and pressure).

iii) The third group, known as disorders of the form of thought, is concerned with abnormalities of the ways in which thoughts are linked together (linking of thoughts together).

iv) The fourth group, abnormal beliefs about the possession of thoughts, comprises unusual disturbances of the normal awareness that one's thoughts are one's own.

i) **Abnormal thoughts (Delusions, obsessions)**
A delusion is a belief that is firmly held on inadequate grounds, is not affected by rational argument or evidence to the contrary and is not a conventional belief.

A delusion is a false unshakable belief.

For the purposes of clinical work, delusions are grouped according to their main themes as follows :

Persecutory delusions are often called paranoid. They are most commonly concerned with persons or organisations that are thought to be trying to inflict harm on the patient, damage his reputation, make him insane, or poison him. They are seen in organic psychosis, schizophrenia and in severe affective disorders.

Delusions of reference (ideas of reference) are concerned with the idea that objects, events or people have a personal significance for the patient. For example, an article read in a newspaper is believed to be directed specifically to himself. This is the commonest symptom seen in paranoid schizophrenia.

Grandiose or expansive delusions are beliefs of exaggerated self-importance. The patient may think himself wealthy, endowed with unusual abilities or a special person. Such ideas occur in mania and in schizophrenia.

Delusion of guilt and worthlessness are found most often in depressive illness and are therefore sometimes called depressive delusions. Typical themes are that a minor infringement of the law in the past will be discovered and bring shame upon the patient or that his sinfulness will lead to divine retribution on his family.

Nihilistic delusions are beliefs about the non-existence of some person or thing. The patient denies the existence of his body, his mind or the world around.

Nihilistic delusions are associated with extreme degrees of depressed mood. Comparable ideas concerning failures of bodily function (e.g. that the bowels are blocked with putrefying matter) often accompany nihilistic delusions.

Hypochondriacal delusions are concerned with illness. The patient may believe wrongly and in the face of all medical evidence to the contrary, that he is ill. Such delusions are more common in the elderly, reflecting the increasing concern with health among normal people at this time of life.

Delusion of jealousy are more common among men. They get preoccupied with obsessional thoughts concerning with doubts about the spouse's fidelity. The doubts may lead to dangerously aggressive behaviour towards the person thought to be unfaithful. A person with delusional jealousy will not be satisfied if he fails to find evidence supporting his beliefs; his search will continue. It is seen in patients with paranoid syndromes.

In **Delusion of control** the patient believes that his actions, impulses or thoughts are controlled by an outside agency. This symptom strongly suggests schizo-phrenia.

ii) Possession of thoughts

Patients with delusions concerning the possession of thoughts may feel that his thoughts are not his own or his thoughts are known to others.

Patients with delusions of thought insertion believe that some of their thoughts are not their own but have been implanted by an outside agency. This experience differs from that of the obsessional patient who may be distressed by unpleasant thoughts but never doubts that they originate within his own mind.

Patients with **delusions of thought withdrawal** believe that thoughts have been taken out of their mind. This delusion usually accompanies thought blocking, so that the patient experiences a break in the flow of thoughts through his mind and believes that the 'missing' thoughts have been taken away by some outside agency, often his supposed persecutors.

Patients with **delusions of thought broadcasting** believe that their unspoken thoughts are known to other people, through radio, telepathy or in some other way.

All three of these symptoms occur much more com-monly in schizophrenia than in any other disorder.

iii) Disorders of stream of thought

In this both the amount and the speed of thoughts are changed.

With pressure of thought the ideas arise in unusual variety and abundance and pass through the mind rapidly. It occurs in Mania.

79

At the other extreme there is **poverty** of thought, when the patient has only a few thoughts, which lack variety and richness and seem to move through the mind slowly. It is seen in depressive disorders. Either may be experienced in schizophrenia.

A sudden, complete and abrupt interruption in the flow of conversation is known as thought block and is seen in schizophrenia.

iv) Disorders of the form of thought

Flight of ideas, where in the patient's thoughts and conversation move quickly from one topic to another. These rapidly changing topics may have a logical sequences of ideas. It is characteristic of mania.

Neologism is an abnormality of speech, wherein the patient uses words or phrases, invented by himself, often to describe his morbid experiences.

Circumstantiality is characterised by thinking proceeding slowly with many unnecessary trivial details but finally the goal is reached. It is seen in mania, organic mental disorders and schizophrenia.

Loosening of associations denotes a loss of the normal structure of thinking. It occurs most often in schizophrenia.

Obsessional symptoms are more common than delusions but generally of less serious significance. Obsessional and compulsive symptoms often occur together.

Obsessions are recurrent, persistent thoughts, impulses or images that enter the mind despite the person's efforts to exclude them.

Compulsions are repetitive and seemingly purposeful behaviour, performed in a stereotyped way. A compulsion is usually associated with an obsession as if it has the function of reducing the distress caused by the latter. For example, a hand washing compulsion often follows obsessional thoughts that the hands are contaminated with faecal matter.

C. Disorders of emotion

The term "affect" is used for short term states, while "mood" for sustained ones. These words are often used interchangeably. In mental illness, affect may be abnormal.

Emotions in mental illness are often changed towards anxiety, depression, elation or anger. Changes in any on these emotions may be associated with an obvious cause in the person's life or arise without reason. Emotional disorders are usually accompanied by autonomic over-activity, increased muscle tension and feelings of depression by gloomy preoccupations and psycho motor slowness.

The fluctuation of mood like **apathy** (without feeling), **blunt** (normal variation of emotion is reduced), **labile** (emotions change in an excessively rapid and abrupt way) and **emotional** incontinence (mood changes are very marked) are often found as symptoms in affective disorders and schizophrenia.

In mental illness, there can be **incongruity** of affect. His thoughts and actions are not congruent with circumstances. For example, a patient may laugh when describing the death of his mother.

Disorders of emotion are found in all kinds of mental illnesses. They form the central feature of the affective

81

disorder (mania and depression) and of anxiety disorders. They are also common in other neuroses, organic disorders and schizophrenia.

D. Disorders of motor activity

Abnormalities of social behaviour, facial expression and posture occur frequently in all mental illnesses.

Tics are irregular repeated movements involving a group of muscles, e.g. sideways movement of the head or the raising of one shoulder. **Mannerisms** are repeated movements that appear to have some functional significance, e.g. saluting. **Stereotypies** are repeated movements that are regular (unlike tics) and without significance (unlike mannerisms), e.g. rocking to and from.

Posturing is the adoption of unusual bodily positions continuously for a long time, e.g. standing on one leg. **Negativism** is that the patient does opposite of what is asked and actively resist efforts to persuade them to comply. **Echopraxia** is the imitation of the interviewer's movement automatically even when asked not to do so. **Echolalia** is the repetition of the interviewer's words. **Waxy flexibility** is detected when a patients limbs can be placed in a position in which they then remain for long periods whilst at the same time muscle tone is uniformly increased.

There are also a number of specific motor symptoms. With the exception of tics all the other symptoms are mainly observed among schizophrenic patients.

E. Disorders of memory

Several kinds of memory failure are seen among psychiatric patients. Patients project a peculiar disturbance of recall, either failing to recognise events that have been encountered before or reporting the recognition of events. Some patients with extreme difficulty in remembering may report as memories, events that have not taken place and/or in which he had no involvement. This is known as confabulation (Filling up of memory gaps with his own ideas).

F. Disorders of consciousness

Consciousness is awareness of the self and the environment. The level of consciousness can vary between the extremes of alertness and coma.

Stupor refers to a condition in which the patient is immobile, mute and unresponsive but appears to be fully conscious. It is seen among schizophrenic patients.

Confusion means the inability to think clearly. It occurs in organic states and in functional disorders.

G. Disorders of attention and concentration

Attention is the focussing one or more sensory organ towards a particular stimulus. Concentration is the ability to maintain that focus. These abilities may be impaired in a wide variety of psychiatric disorders including depressive disorders, mania, anxiety disorders, schizophrenia and organic disorders.

H. Insight

It may be defined as awareness of one's own mental condition. Patients being aware of their behavioural disturbances and seeking treatment for the same refers to 'insight present'. Neurosis is a minor mental illness in which insight is present. Psychosis is a major mental illness in which insight is absent. 'Insight' is considered to be one of the important criteria to diagnose a patient whether he is psychotic or neurotic.

Questions

1. How do you explain the concept of normalcy and abnormalcy in human behaviour?

2. Discuss the features of disturbances of mental illness in bodily functions.

3. Write short notes on :

   i)   Medical model

   ii) Statistical model

   iii) Socio-cultural model

4. How do you classify mental disorders?

5. Write short notes on :

   i)   ICD-10

   ii) DSM

   iii) Indian classification of mental illness

   iv) Psychosis

   v)   Neurosis

   vi) Mental retardation

6. Enumarate signs and symptoms of major mental illness.

7. Write short notes on :

   i)   Insight

ii) Disorders of thought

iii) Hallucination

8. Define the following terms :

i) Echolalia

ii) Echopraxia

iii) Circumstantiality

iv) Flight of ideas

v) Nihilistic delusion

vi) Delusion of grandiosity

vii) Waxy flexibility

viii) Illusion

ix) Delusion

x) Obsessive-compulsive behaviour

9. Outline the mental status examination of a psychiatric patient.

MANAGEMENT

Drug Therapy

The advent of psychotropic medication has generated dramatic results in the treatment of the mentally ill. The nurse needs to understand the importance and usefulness of these medications. Recognising the desired actions, adverse reactions of the drugs, normal therapeutic dosages, documenting medication administration and keeping abreast of current literature on the psychotropic drugs are some of the responsibilities of the nurse.

To understand psychopharmacology, nurses must understand two concepts - neurotransmitters and the blood-brain barrier.

Neurotransmitters

Nerve cells or neurones are the basic unit of the nervous system. They receive and give information. Dendrites are the projections from the neuron that receive information and transmit it to the cell body. Axons send information from the nerve cell to the dendrites of other neurones. Axons of one cell are separated from the dendrites of another by a microscopic space known as a synapse.

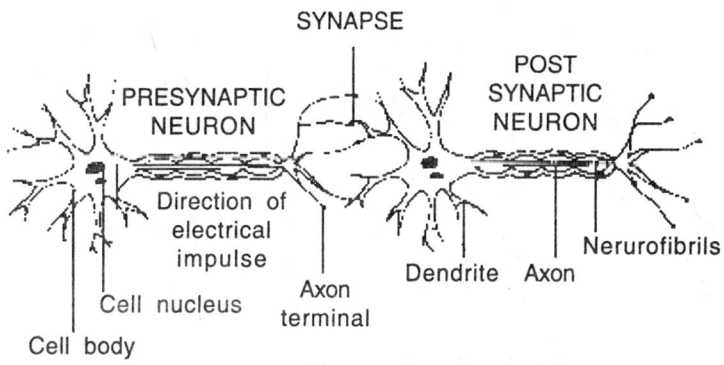

Neurotransmitter precursors produced in the cell body are carried by neurofibrils to axon terminals cuases release of neurotransmitters at synapse.

The synapse separates two neurones (the pre-synaptic cell and the post-synaptic cell) at a transmission site. During neurotransmission, the chemical neurotransmitter is released from a storage vehicle in the pre-synaptic cell, crosses the synapse, and is recognised by the receptor on the post-synaptic cell membrane (this recognition is called binding). Receptors are the cellular recognition sites for specific molecular structures such as neurotransmitters, hormones and many drugs. Thus their action is selective for specific chemicals.

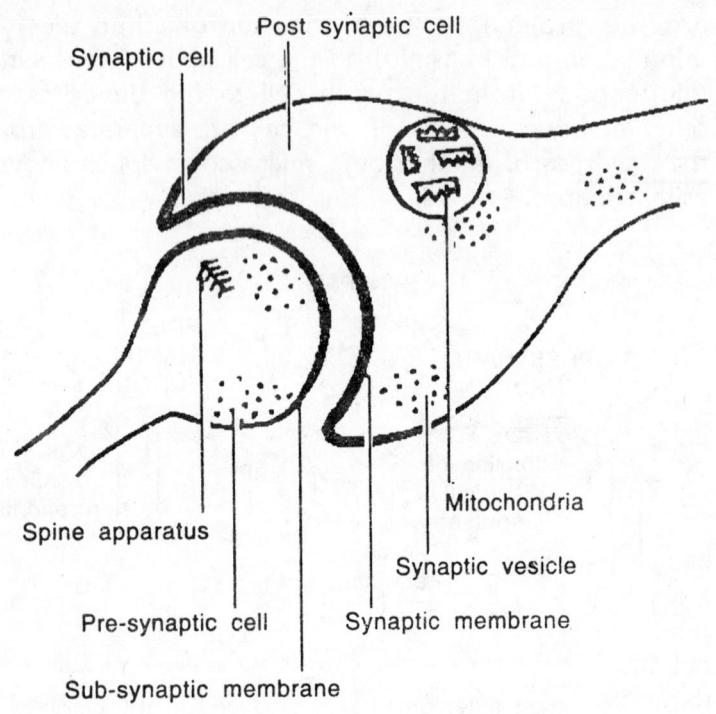

Post synaptic cell

Synaptic cell

Spine apparatus

Pre-synaptic cell

Sub-synaptic membrane

Mitochondria

Synaptic vesicle

Synaptic membrane

An axodendrite synapse

Neurotransmitters, the "chemical messengers" that travel from one brain cell to another, are synthesised by enzymes from certain dietary amino acids, or precursors. At the synapse, neurotransmitters act as receptor activators (agonists) or inhibitors (antagonists) and bigger complex biological responses within the cell. The chemical remaining in the synapse is either reabsorbed and stored by the pre-synaptic cell or is metabolised (inactivated) by synaptic enzymes, one of which is monoamine oxidase.

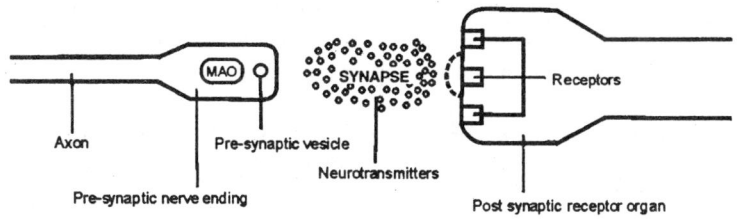

Axon   Pre-synaptic vesicle

Neurotransmitters

Pre-synaptic nerve ending   Post synaptic receptor organ

Neurotransmission at the synapse

Many of the psychiatric disorders are thought to be caused by an over-response or an under-response somewhere along the complex process of neurotransmission. Psychosis is thought to involve excessive dopamine neurotransmission. Depression and Mania are thought to result from disruption of normal patterns of neuro transmission of norepinephrine, serotonin and other neurotransmitters. Anxiety is thought to be a dysregulation of gamma-amino butyric acid (GABA) and endogenous anti-anxiety chemicals.

The drugs affect the process of neurotransmission at the synapse in several ways:

(i)   **release** : more neurotransmitter is released into the synapse from the storage vesicles in the pre-synaptic cell.

(ii)   **blockade** : the neurotransmitters are prevented from binding to the post-synaptic receptor.

(iii) **receptor sensitivity changes** : the receptor becomes more or less responsive to the neurotransmitter.

(iv) **blocked re-uptake** : the pre-synaptic cell does not reabsorb the neurotransmitter well, leaving more neurotransmitter in the synapse and therefore enhancing or prolonging its action.

(v) **interference with storage vesicles** : the neurotransmitter is either released more or released less.

(vi) **precursor chain interference** : the process that "makes" the neurotransmitter is more synthesised or less.

(vii) **synaptic enzyme interference** : less neurotransmitter is metabolised, so more remains available in the synapse.

Antipsychotic drugs block dopamine from the receptor site; tricyclic antidepressants block the re-uptake of norepinephrine and serotonin and regulate the areas of the brain that manufacture these chemicals; monoamine oxidase inhibitors prevent enzymatic metabolism of norepinephrine and serotinin; and benzodiazepines potentiate GABA. Chemotherapy in psychiatry is based on this knowledge of transmitters or, in other words, the pharmacotherapy is based on the knowledge of this pathology. The drugs used in psychiatry are classified according to action of the drug on the nerve cell, that is on the neurotransmitters either by increasing or decreasing the secretion or absorption.

Psychotropic drug classification

Drugs that have effects mainly on mental symptoms are called psychotropic. They are classified as follows:

90

I. Antidepressants

(i)   tricyclic antidepressant (TCA)

(ii) monoamine oxidase inhibitor (MAOI)

(iii) tetracyclic antidepressant

II. Antimanics

III. Benzodiazepines

IV. Antipsychotics

V. Psychostimulants

VI. Antiparkinsonian agents

VII. Miscellaneous agents

I. Antidepressants

It is believed that antidepressants block the re-uptake of various neurotransmitters, especially dopamine, serotonin and norepinephrine at the neural synapse. They show strong anticholinergic action. The effect of norepinephrine and serotinin are the principle ones. TCA may lower the seizure threshold and increase alpha activity.

Pharmacokinetics : Absorbs from G. I. tract. Distribution – they and their metabolics are bound to plasma proteins and tissue protein. They cross placenta and breast milk. Elimination : Metabolised in liver. They cross the brain barrier.

Drugs used as TCA

Amitriptyline, Doxepin, Imipramine, Trimipramine.

Side effects

Autonomic : Dry mouth, disturbance of accommodation, difficult micturation leading to retention, constipation leading rarely to ileus, postural hypotension, tachycardia and increased sweating.

Psychiatric : Tiredness and drowsiness, insomnia (with imipramine). Acute organic syndromes and mania may be provoked in manic depressive patients.

Cardiovascular effects : Tachycardia, hypotension, changes in E.C.G.

Neurological : Fine tremors, incoordination, headache, muscle twitch, epileptic seizures in predisposed patients and peripheral neuropathy.

Other : Allergic skin rashes, mild jaundice and rarely agranulocytosis.

Antidepressants should be withdrawn slowly. Sudden cessation may be followed by nausea, anxiety, sweating and insomnia.

M.A.O.I.

It is an enzyme which catalyses the re-uptake of norepinephrine, serotonin and dopamine. The inhibition of enzyme produces increased concentration of these amines in nerve tissue and in the liver and lungs.

Drugs used

Isocarboxazid, Phenelzine

Side effects

Postural hypotension, constipation, muscle twitch, dry mouth, fluid retention, insomnia, urinary hesitancy.

II. Antimanics

Sodium metabolism within nerves and muscles enhances the re-uptake of biogenic amines in the brain, and lowers the level of amines in the body, resulting in decreased hyperactivity. Antimanics also have antidepressive activity. They are called as "mood stabilisers".

Pharmacokinetics

The drug is rapidly absorbed from G. I. tract and quickly go throughout the body fluids interfering with the magnesium and calcium. Elimination: It moves out of cells slowly. It is removed from plasma by renal excretion.

Distribution

It is found in extracellular fluid and breast milk.

Drugs used

Lithium carbonate, Carbomazapine.

(i) Lithium Salts

As a treatment for mania, lithium salts where first employed in 1949 by Cade in Australia. The principal use of lithium is to prevent recurrence of mania, depressive disorders and acute episodes of mania.

Lithium is rapidly absorbed from the gut and diffuses quickly throughout the body fluids and cells, displacing sodium and potassium and interfering with maganesium and calcium. Lithium moves out of cells more slowly than sodium. It is removed from plasma by renal excretion and by entering cells and other body compartments. There is, therefore, a rapid excretion of lithium from the plasma, and a slower phase reflecting its removal from the whole body pool. Lithium, like sodium, is filtered and partly reabsorbed in the kidney. When the proximal tubule absorbs more water, lithium absorption increases. Therefore, dehydration causes plasma lithium concentration to rise. Because lithium is transported in competition with sodium, more is reabsorbed when sodium concentration falls. Thiazide diuretics increase sodium excretion without increasing that of lithium; hence they can lead to toxic concentrations of lithium in the blood.

Contra indication

Cardiac vascular disease, severe renal disease, severe dehydration, pregnancy, lactation, hypothyroidism, history of seizure.

Side effects

C.N.S : Confusion, dizziness, weakness, headache, lethargy.

C.V.S : Arrhythmias, hypotension, ECG changes.

Dermatology : Drying and thinning of hair.

Endocrine : Hypothyrodism.

G.I. tract : Anorexia, nausea, vomiting, diarrhoea, dry mouth, thirst.

G. U. tract: Polyuria, Glucosuria, diabetes insepedus oliguria.

Haematology : Irreversible leukocytosis.

Pharmacokinetics

Absorption : Through G.I. tract.

Distribution : Widely distributed. It is found in cerebro spinal fluid, plasma and crosses placental barrier and found in breast milk.

Metabolism : Not metabolised and found in body as such.

Excretion : Excreted in urine.

Interaction with drugs

Aminophylline, Manitol and drugs rich in sodium will decrease the effectiveness of lithium. Phenothiazines decrease the antipsychotic effect or increased lithium excretion.

Interaction with food

Increased dietary intake of sodium will increase renal elimination of lithium. Decreased dietary intake will cause retention of lithium and lead to toxicity.

Toxic effects

Ataxia, poor concentration of limb movements, muscle twitch, slurred speech and confusion. They constitute a serious medical emergency, for they can progress through coma and fits to death. If these symptoms appear, lithium must be stopped at once and a high intake of fluid should be provided with extra sodium chloride to stimulate and increase osmotic diuresis. In severe cases renal dialysis may be needed. Lithium is rapidly cleared, if renal function is normal. So that the most cases either recover completely or die. However, a few cases of permanent neurological damage despite haemodialysis have been reported.

Lithium crosses the placenta and causes abnormalities in the babies of mothers receiving lithium in pregnancy. Lithium is also secreted into breast milk. Therefore lithium should be avoided in the first trimester of pregnancy and bottle feeding is a wise distribution.

Management

Before starting lithium

A physical examination should be carried out. Blood pressure, weight, urine for protein, sugar and casts, eletrolytes, urea, serum creatinine, Hb, ESR, blood count, and thyroid function test to be done. If indicated, ECG, pregnancy tests, or lithium clearance should be done. A careful explanation should be given, and make sure that the patient is not taking a thiazide diuretics.

After starting

Treatment should begin and continue with two doses 12 hours apart. If the drug is being used for prophylaxis, it is appropriate to begin with 750 – 1000 mg per day in divided doses, taking blood for lithium estimations every week and adjusting the dose until an appropriate concentration is achieved. For prophylaxis, a lithium level of 0.4 to 0.8 mmol/1 (in a sample taken 12 hours after the last dose) may be adequate, as explained above; if this is not effective, the high range of 0.7 to 1.2 mmol/1 should be used.

While on treatment

Lithium estimation should be carried out every six weeks. Every six months, blood sample should be taken for electrolytes, urea, creatinine, a full blood count, and thyroid function test. Special care to be taken before starting Halophidol or any other antipsychotic drug, ECT and anaesthesia.

Lithium is usually continued for at least a year and may continue for not more than five years. When lithium is withdrawn suddenly, some patients become irritable and emotionally labile, and a few relapse into mania. It is prudent to withdrawn lithium gradually.

(ii) Carbomezapine (Tegretol)

Action	: Not fully known, but believed to be mood stabiliser and anticonvulsant.
Absorption	: From G.I. tract.
Distribution	: Crosses blood barrier and placental barrier, and excreted in breast milk.
Metabolism	: In liver and excreted by kidneys.

Contra indication : T.C.A, MAOI, lactation and bone while patient is on, marrow depression.

Side effects

C.N.S : Drowsiness, confusion, headache, ataxia.

C.V.S : Hypertension, arrhythemia.

Dermatology : Rashes, urticaria, pigmentation.

G.I.T : Nausea, vomiting, diarrhoea, dry mouth, abdominal pain.

Others : Jaundice, hepatitis.

Route and dosage : Oral preparation upto 1.2 gm/day.

Repeat plasma levels to see the toxicity. Normal level is 3 to 14 mg/ml.

III. Benzodiazepines

Action : Acts on nervous system potentially by inhibiting few neurotransmitters. It has anxiolytic, hypnotic, sedative, antoconvulsant and muscle relaxant properties.

The pharmacological action is located in supramolecular complex with GABA (gamma amino butyric acid) receptors. They enhance GABA neurotransmission, thereby altering indirectly the activity of other neurotransmitter systems such as those involving noradrenaline.

Pharmacokinetics

Rapidly absorbed, bound to plasma protein. Excretion is mainly as conjugates in the urine.

Drugs used

Lorazepam, Diazepam, Oxazepam, Alprozolam, Alprax, Alepax, Librium.

Side effects

It starts from drowsiness to cardiac arrest.

Give slowly if administered intravenously. Check the vital signs every 5 minutes for 1 hour. While discontinuing the treatment, withdraw slowly to prevent withdrawal symptoms like sleeplessness, headache, tension and anxiety.

IV. Antipsychotics

Antipsychotic agents control some of the symptoms of schizophrenia, mania and organic psychoses. The term antipsychotics is applied to drugs that reduce psychomotor excitement and control some symptoms of schizophrenia without causing disinhibition confusion or sleep. Alternative terms for these drugs are neuroleptic, antischizophrenic and major tranquillizer.

The main therapeutic uses of antipsychotics are to reduce hallucinations, delusions, agitations and psychomotor excitement in schizophrenia, organic psychosis or mania. These drugs are also used prophylactically to prevent relapses of schizophrenia. In 1952, the introduction of chlorpromazine led to substantial improvements in the treatment of schizophrenia and paved the way to the discovery of many psychotropic drugs now available.

Pharmacology

They share the property of blocking dopamine receptors. This may account for therapeutic action. Alpha isomer block dopamine receptors and is therapeutic, while beta isomer does not block dopamine receptors and is not therapeutic. Both Alpha and Beta isomers block noradrenergic and cholenergic receptors. The antiadrenergic actions account for many side effects of the drug, while antidopaminergic actions on basal ganglia are responsible for the EPS (extra pyramidal symptoms).

Pharmacokinetics

Well absorbed, mainly from jejunum. Metabolised in liver. Combinations of active and inactive metabolites also occur with other antipsychotic drugs. Excreted through urine. Stored in the fat. Even after stopping the drug, action continues because of slow elimination.

Side effects

The many different antipsychotic drugs share a broad pattern of unwanted effects that are mainly related to their antidopaminergic, antiadrenergic and anticholinergic properties.

Extrapyramidal effects

These are related to the antidopaminergic action of the drugs of the basal ganglia. The effects of the extrapyramidal system fall into four groups.

(i)   Acute dystonia

It occurs soon after treatment begins, specially in young men. It is observed most often with butyrophenones

100

and with the piperazine group of phenothiazines. The main features are torticollis, tongue protrusion, grimacing and opisthotonus, an odd clinical picture wh ich can easily be mistaken for histrionic behaviour It can be controlled by biperiden lactate 2 to 5 mg, given carefully by intramuscular injection or in the most severe cases, by slow intravenous injection.

(ii) Akathisia

It is an unpleasant feeling of physical restlessness and need to move, lead to an inability to keep still. It occurs usually in the first two weeks of treatment with neuroleptic drugs, but may begin only after several months. Akathisia is not controlled by antiparkinsonian drugs, but when occuring early in treatment it disappears if the dose is reduced. Occassional late cases have been described which do not respond quickly to a reduction in dose. It is difficult to differenciate these cases from tardive dyskinesia.

(iii) Parkinsonian syndrome

This is the common side effects characterised by akinesia – an expressionless face and lack of associated movements when walking, together with rigidity, tremor, stooped posture and in, severe cases, a festinant gait. This syndrome often takes a few weeks to appear after the drug has been taken and then sometimes diminishes, even though the doses have not been reduced. The symptoms can be controlled with antiparkinsonian drugs. However, it is not a good practice to prescribe antiparkinsonian drugs prophylactically as a routine, because not all the patients will need them.

101

Moreover, these drugs themselves have undesirable effects in some patients, e.g., they occasionally cause an acute organic syndrome, and possibly increase the incidence of tardive dyskinesia.

(iv) Tardive dyskinesia

The last syndrome, tardive dyskinesia, is particularly serious because, unlike the other extrapyramidal effects, it does not always recover when the drugs are stopped. It is characterised by chewing and sucking movements, grimacing, choreothetoid movements and possibly akathisia. The last mentioned usually affect the face but the limbs and the muscles of respiration may also be involved. Tardive dyskinesia is more common among women, the elderly and the patients who have diffused brain pathology. In about half the cases, tardive dyskinesia disappears when the drugs are stopped. Estimates of the frequency of the syndrome in different series, but it seems to develop in 20-40 percent of schizophrenic patients treated with long-term antipsychotic drugs.

The cause of the syndrome is uncertain but it could possibly be supersensitivity to dopamine resulting from prolonged dopaminergic blockade.

Many treatments for tardive dyskinesia have been tried, but none is universally effective. It is important, therefore, to reduce its incidence as far as possible by limiting long-term treatment and high doses to patients who really need them. At the same time, a careful watch should be kept for abnormal movements in all patients who have taken antipsychotic drugs for a long time.

If dyskinesia is observed, the antipsychotic drug should be stopped, if the state of mental illness allows this.

Although dyskinesia may at first worsen after stopping the drug, in many cases it will improve over several months. If the continuation of antipsychotic medication is essential, haloperidol, pimozide and dopamine depleting agents such as tetrabenazine can be administered.

Antiadrenergic effects

These include postural hypotension with tachycardia, nasal congestion, and inhibition of ejaculation. The effects on blood pressure are likely to appear after intramuscular administration, and in the elderly whatever the route of administration.

Anticholinergic effects

These include dry mouth, urinary retention, constipation, reduced sweating, blurred vision and rarely the precipitation of glaucoma.

Other effects

Arrythmias, changes in ECG, depression of mood, weight gain, galactorrhoea, amenorrhoea, hypothermia specially in elderly, seizures in epileptic patients, photo sensitivity and accumulation of pigment in the skin, cornea and lens. Thioridazine in exceptionally high doses (more than 800 mg/day) may cause retinal degeneration. Rare adverse reactions include cholestatic jaundice and agranulocytosis.

The neuroleptic malignant syndrome

This is a rare but serious disorder that occurs in a small minority of patients taking neuroleptics, especially high potency compound. The clinical picture includes the rapid onset (usually over 24-72 hours) of severe motor, mental and autonomic disorders. The prominent motor symptom is muscular hypertonicity. Stiffness of the muscles in the throat and chest may cause dysphagia and dyspnoea. The mental symptoms include akinetic mutism, stupor and impaired consciousness. Hyperpyrexia develops with evidence of autonomic disturbances in the form of unstable blood pressure, tachycardia, excessive sweating, salivation, and urinary incontinence. In the blood, creatinine phosphokinase (CPK) levels may be raised, and the white cells increased. Secondary features may include preumonia, thromboembolism, cardio-vascular collapse and renal failure. The syndrome lasts for one or two weeks after stopping an oral neuroleptics. Patients who survive are without residual disability.

The treatment is symptomatic. The main needs are to stop the drugs, cool the patient, maintain fluid balance, and treat intercurrent infection. No single drug treatment is fully effective. Diazepam can be used for muscle stiffness. Dantrolene, a drug used to treat malignant hyperthermia, has also been tried. Bromocriptine, amantadine and L-dopa have been used but with insufficient cases for a definite statement about their value. Some patients who developed the syndrome on one occasion have been given the drug safely after the acute episode has resolved.

Drugs used

There are five categories of antipsychotic drugs. They are:

1. Phenothiazines   : Chlorpromazine, Thioridazine, Mesoridazine, Perphenazine, Trifluoperazine, Fluphenazine

2. Thioxanthene : Thiothixene

3. Butyrophenone : Haloperidol, Pimozide

4. Dibenzoxazepine : Loxapine

5. Dihydroindolone : Molindone

An atypical category is Dibenzodiazepine. The drug available in this group is clozapine.

(V) Psychostimulants

This class of drugs includes mild stimulants. The best known is caffeine, fencamfamin, meclofenoxate, and pemoline. These mild stimulants are advocated for the treatment of states of fatigue and senility. They are not suitable for the treatment of depressive disorders.

The most important of the powerful stimulants are the amphetamines. But they give rise to dependence. They are not appropriate for the treatment of depressive disorders. They are used in the treatment of narcolepsy.

The main preparations are dexamphetamine sulphate, given for narcolepsy in divided doses of 10 mg per day increasing to a maximum of 50 mg/day by steps of 10 mg each week, and methylamphetamine hydrochloride which has similar effects.

Side effects

These include restlessness, insomnia, poor appetite, dizziness, tremor, palpitations and cardiac arrhythmias. Toxic effects from large doses include disorientation and aggressive behaviour, hallucinations, convulsions and coma. Persistant abuse can lead to a paranoid state similar to paranoid schizophrenia. Amphetamines interact dangerously with monoamine oxidase inhibitors. They are contra indicated in cardiovascular disease and thyrotoxicosis.

VI. Antiparkinsonian agents

They are used to control the extrapyramidal side effects of antipsychotic drugs.

Pharmacology

Of the drugs used to treat idiopathic parkinsonism, the anticholinergic compounds are used for drug-induced extrapyramidal syndromes.

Drugs used

The drugs often used in psychiatric practice are the synthetic anticholinergics, benzhexol, benztropine mesylate and procyclidine; and the antihistaminic, orphenadrine. Orphenadrine is said to have a mood elevating effect. An injectable preparation of biperiden is useful for the treatment of acute dystonias.

Side effects

Acute organic syndrome, specially in elderly, glaucoma, retention of urine in men with enlarged prostates. Drowsiness, dry mouth and constipation also occur. These effects tend to diminish as the drug is continued. There is some evidence that these drugs, when used for prolonged antipsychotic treatment, increase the likelihood of tardive dyskinesia.

VII. Miscellaneous agents

Under this classification, mainly antiepileptic drugs are discussed. Antiepileptic drugs are also called as anticonvulsants. The drugs are usually given prophylactically. A single seizure is not treated. When seizures are continuous (status epilepticus) or frequently repeated with recovery in between (serial seizures) drugs are needed to arrest the condition.

Drugs used

Hydantoins, barbiturates, succinimides, benzodiazepines, carbamazepine and sodium valporate.

Pharmacokinetics

Phenobarbitone increases seizure threshold whereas phenytoin appears to limit the propagation of the discharge.

Most are readily absorbed except phenytoin. They are metabolised in liver and excreted in the urine.

Side effects

All antiepileptic drugs are potentially harmful and must be used with care.

Phenytoin has many adverse effects, gum hypertrophy, acne, hirsutism and coarsening of the facial features. Ataxia, dysarthria, nystagmus, intoxication, high plasma concentration, encephalopathy and uncommon haematological effect.

Carbamazepine has fewer unwanted effects. Drowsiness, ataxia and diplopia develop if the plasma concentration is too high; erythematous rash, water retention, hepatitis, leucopaenia or other blood dyscrasias.

Sodium valporate has few adverse effects like gastrointestinal disturbance (often prevented by taking the drug with food, or by taking an enteric-coated preparation) obesity, thrombocytopenia, tremor, transient hair loss, and serious impairment of liver function.

The unwanted effects of phenobarbitone includes drowsiness, irritability, slurred speech and ataxia. In children hyperactivity and emotional upset are frequent and impaired learning and skin rashes can occur.

Questions

1.   How do you classify psychotropic drugs?

2.   Write short notes on :

   i)   Neuro chemical transmitters

   ii)   Classification of anti-depressants

   iii) Antimanics

   iv)   Management of patient on Lithium

   v)   Side effects of carbomezapine

   vi)   Extrapyramidal symptoms

   vii) Neuroleptic malignant syndrome

viii)   Antiparkinsonian drugs

ix)   Largactil

x)   MAOI

xi)   Benzodiazepines

Physical Therapy

Narco-analysis

Somatic therapies are treatment approaches that use physiological or physical interventions to effect behavioural change. The most common form of somatic therapy is Electroconvulsive Therapy (ECT) and the less common somatic therapy approach is narcotherapy/narco-analysis.

The term "narcotherapy" refers to the intravenous injection of drugs into the patient, as an adjunct to psychotherapy. The induction of a state of sedation by intravenous administration of sedatives (e.g. amobarbital) or stimulants (e.g., methylphenidate) to the patient to become more amenable to psychotherapeutic intervention.

Purpose

The creation of an altered state of awareness or consciousness will facilitate the diagnosis and treatment of psychiatric illnesses.

During the procedure, traumatic events are re-experienced, and the unconscious emotions associated with the events are expressed. Interpretation of information about traumatic or repressed experiences assists the treatment team as they formulate appropriate intervention strategies.

110

History

Blackwenn was the first to advocate the intravenous injection of sodium amytal in psychiatric conditions. Subsequently, in 1926, Horsley originated the "narcoanalysis", which involved the use of both sodium pentothal and sodium amytal.

Techniques

The use of intravenous injections of barbiturates may vary in terms of procedures involved, which, inturn, will depend on the specific treatment goals. Essentially, three techniques are utilised in narcotherapy which may be described as follows:

(i) Simple catharsis

The use of the pentothal interview simply to facilitate catharsis is the technique used least frequently. In addition, it is probably the least effective application of narcotherapy. In brief, the disturbing conflict is elicited with affect (abreaction). However, the material uncovered is not adequately integrated into the total personality. Consequently, while the experience may be effective, its long-term results are relatively unpredictable.

(ii) Suggestion

The therapist makes suggestions to the patient while he is under the influence of the drug, without attempting to uncover repressed material. Thus, this technique resembles supportive psychotherapy, and, as is true of all treatment procedures based on suggestion, while it may have some temporary value, the ability of the patient to maintain his therapeutic gains is questionable.

111

(iii) Narco-analysis and narco synthesis

Both these procedures involve the subsequent application of psychotherapeutic techniques to help the patient integrate and work through the material that has been elicited through the use of the drug.

Narco-analysis through pentothal

The pentothal interview helps the patient to establish a relationship with the therapist, which may be the first step in altering his view of the world and his environment, so that he no longer sees these as completely hostile forces in relation to his needs and desires.

More specifically, the patient's illness and symptoms serve as a protection against the breakthrough of the anxiety which surrounds his underlying conflicts. The drug appears to lessen this anxiety so that the patient can better tolerate expression of painful psychic material. This expression, in turn, facilitates the process of exploration.

In some patients, the drug seems to produce a mild euphoria and to weaken inhibiting mechanisms as well. In any event, the overall effect of the pentothal injection is to enable the patient to tolerate painful insights, and to incorporate them into his emotional and intellectual life.

Dosage

Sodium pentothal is marked for intravenous use in the form of sterile powder in ampules of varying strength. Pentothal solutions are used in concentrations ranging from 2.5 to 5 percent. Usually, the dosage required for satisfactory narcosis varies between 0.25 and 0.5 gm, although more than 1.0 gm may be necessary for larger individuals in extreme states of agitation. As might be expected, the effect of the drug will vary, at least to some extent, with the strength of the concentration of the pentothal solution, the dosage administered, and the rate of injection. In addition, other variables, such as the patient's age, weight, previous food intake, previous barbiturate ingestion, and his cross-tolerance to other sedatives (for example, glutethimide) will also influence the effect of the drug.

Administration

Before administering the drug, the physician should establish a positive rapport with the patient. More specifically, the patient is told that the drug will help him to relax and feel more at ease, and that it will permit him to talk more freely and comfortably about the feelings and experiences that bother him. Concomitantly, the common misconception that pentathol is a magic truth serum should be dispelled.

The drug is best administered in a quiet room, with the patient in a reclining position. The injection is made into an antecubital vein. When the 5 percent pentothal solution is used, the injection is made at the rate of 2 cc per minute. When the weaker solution is used, the injection is made at a more rapid rate. During the injection, the patient may complain of a peculiar taste in his mouth; in addition, in many instances, there is some initial increase in anxiety or agitation.. However, as the injection continues, these symptoms tend to disappear.

At the outset, and until the physician becomes familiar with the patient's characteristic response to the drug, it is best to ask him to count backward from 100 immediately after the injection is made. Shortly after counting becomes confused, but before the patient actually falls asleep, the injection is stopped. It is at this point that psychological interaction between patient and therapist occurs. It is at this point that attempts are made to discuss significant material, to elicit repressed experiential data, or to make appropriate suggestions. The patient is then permitted to go to sleep.

Indications

Narco-analysis may provide symptomatic relief for severely agitated patients. Where psychotherapeutic exploration seems blocked, it may constitute a new therapeutic approach. The effect of pentothal injections may, of course, be quite dramatic in case of hysterical amnesia.

The treatment provides opportunity to ventilate the significant life experiences which played a vital etiological role in the patient's illness.

The pentothal interview may be used as a diagnostic and prognostic tool as well. The injection may elicit suicidal or paranoid ideas which might not be detected otherwise. It can be used in differential diagnosis to help distinguish organic disabilities from functional syndromes. And it may also be used as a test for organic brain disease, in as much as it provokes neurological symptoms which may not be apparent under "normal" conditions. In addition, in the course of the interview, such mental symptoms as confabulation, disorientation

114

and denial of illness, which may not have been apparent previously, frequently emerge in response to direct questioning.

On occasion, the drug has aided in the differential diagnosis between the catatonic stupor of schizophrenia and stuporous depressive state. Ordinarily, it is difficult to differentiate between these psychopathological entities on the basis of clinical data. The pentothal interview has led to the formulation of specific criteria to facilitate such differentiation. In the depressed patient an intravenous injection of barbiturate will usually result in a deepening of the stupor and/or sleep. In schizophrenic patients with catatonic stupor, such an injection often produces a temporary clearing of the stupor, during which the patient may communicate rationally with the therapist, at least briefly.

Finally, the pentathol interview has also been used in legal investigations. However, the present consensus is that there is no certainty that the subject will "confess" under the influence of the drug, or, if he does, that his account will be accurate. Moreover, the courts have adopted a rather paradoxial attitude towards this procedure. Information obtained by this procedure is not admitted as legal evidence, though the psychiatric implications of such data does carry considerable weight.

Contra indications

Intravenous pentothal injections are contra indicated in the presence of any medical illness which would contra indicate the use of barbiturate, e.g., severe cardiac impairment, porphyria, kidney dysfunction, or liver pathology. General disability, marked emaciation or severe anaemias are other reliable contra indications. Finally, for the most part, the procedure should be limited to adults.

Post-procedural care

When milder doses of pentothal drug is administered to an ambulatory patient, the patient should be permitted to rest after the interview and should not leave the physician's office/treatment room unaccompanied.

It should also be borne in mind that the pentothal induced narco-analysis is not an isolated treatment. No matter how limited (or extensive) the physician's goal is, the psychiatrist who conduct the analysis must have a fundamental knowledge of the psychodynamics of his patient's emotional and mental functioning.

Questions

1. Define narco-analysis.

2. Specify the purpose of doing narco-analysis.

3. Discuss the techniques used in narco-analysis.

4. Identify the indications and contra indications of doing narco-analysis.

5. How will you assist the psychiatrist for the procedure of narco-analysis?

116

Shock Therapy

Explosion in knowledge and the impact of science and technology is being felt in all walks of life. Its impact is greatly felt in medical science wherein more complicated instruments have been designed and used in various types of diseases. One such instrument used in treating mental illness is Electro Convulsive Therapy (ECT).

Ladislas Van Meduna used the convulsant agent to treat schizophrenic patients. After an extensive research for suitable convulsant agent Meduna selected camphor in oil. On January 23, 1934 in the state hospital at Budapest, Meduna gave the first injection of camphor to a male catatonic schizophrenic patient. He later switched to more reliable convulsant drug like cardiozol. It is because that his neuropathological studies on the epileptic patients gave an observation of crushing growth of glial cells in the brains, in contrast to lack of glial reactions in the brains of schizophrenic patients. At the same time, international league against epilepsy released a mono-graph about producing artificial convulsions with cam-phor-monobromide. That made Meduna to use camphor to produce experimental epilepsy on guinea pigs. Later he injected camphor in oil to a catatonic schizophrenic stupor patient who never moved, never ate, remained incontinent and required tube feeding for four years.

117

Within 45 minutes of injection the patient had a classical epileptic attack for 60 seconds and showed full recovery. Meduna published his results in a sample of 26 schizophrenic patients : 10 recovered, three had good results, and 13 did not respond. Then Meduna replaced camphor with the chemically related pentylentetrrazol (cardiazol, metrazol), because of its solubility and rapid onset of action.

Drug induced convulsions were expensive, unreliable and unpleasant to the patients. Working from 1936, Cerletti and Bini attempted to develop safe standards for the use of electricity as an alternative to induce therapeutic convulsions in mentally ill patients. Whereas in 1934, Chiauzzi had produced seizure in dogs by passing a 50-Hz 220-V stimulus for 0.25 second across electrodes placed in the mouth and rectum. Bini found the danger of passing current through oral-rectal electrodes with heart lying in the path of electricity. He demonstrated the safety of applying both the electrodes to the temple of the dogs.

At Rome, the electrical stimulus was applied to the heads of pigs to produce convulsion. The applicators were removed while the pigs were comatosed. It proved that transcerebral electrical stimulation did not kill the pigs. Hence, continued attempts were made by Cerletti and Bini to refine the electrical stimulus parameters that might be safe and effective for human application.

In April 1938, Bini and Cerletti in Rome for the first time administered ECT to a man of 39 years old, a wandering lunatic. He was alternating between periods of mutism and incomprehensible, neologistic speech and was hallucinating. The first shock "stunned" the patient, but was sub-convulsive (70 V for 0.2 second). Cerletti

118

repeated the treatment at higher voltage (100 V) and successfully induced a convulsion with uneventful recovery.

Since its introduction ECT has proved to be an effective treatment for some psychiatric disorders, especially as the treatment of choice for patients with psychotic or endogenous depression.

However, ECT has remained controversial, considered by the public and by some psychiatrists as non-therapeutic or even harmful. This is due to the misrepresentation of ECT as "shock" therapy or treatment.

It was projected as punitive, noxious and oldfashioned, in total disregard to its merits. Treating psychiatric patients with ECT was also considered as barbaric and dangerous and therefore revolting.

From 1980 onwards, ECT is being considered as a unique psychiatric, treatment requiring general anaesthesia, and nurse's role in this therapy has become indispensible.

Definition

Electroconvulsive therapy is a type of somatic treatment in which electric current is applied to the brain through electrodes placed on the temples of the patient. The passage of an electrical stimulus of 70 to 150 volts to the brain for 0.1 to 0.5 second to produce a grandmal seizure. The amount of voltage and the length of application vary with each client. The dosage is adjusted to the minimal amount of electrical current necessary to produce a seizure. Individual seizure thresholds vary, and are generally found to be higher in females and older people.

Mechanism of action

The exact mechanism is unknown. But it is thought to produce biochemical changes in the brain – an increase in the levels of norephinephrine and serotonin – similar to the effects of antidepressant medications.

ECT device

The apparatus used to convert the AC main supply (sinewave) into stimulus uses a step-down transformer to yield a choice of voltage ranging from 70 V to 180 V in steps of 10 volts. The stimulus duration can be chosen from 0.1 sec to 1.0 sec in steps of 0.1 sec each or (rarely) longer. The apparatus offers facilities to read the voltage as well as current delivered during the stimulus administration.

Indications

ECT is indicated for patients with the diagnosis of psychotic depression, mania, catatonia and schizophrenia.

ECT is primarily used in the treatment of severe depression. It is sometimes administered in conjunction with antidepressant medication, but most physicians prefer to perform this treatment only after an unsuccessful trial of drug therapy.

ECT may also be used as a fast-acting treatment for very hyperactive manic patients in danger of physical exhaustion, and for individuals who are extremely suicidal.

There has been evidences, however, of its effectiveness in the treatment of acute psychoses and catatonia.

ECT is preferred to antidepressant therapy in some cases, such as for clients with heart conditions, for whom tricyclics are contra indicated because of the potential for dysrythmia and congestive heart failure, and for pregnant women, in whom antidepressants place the foetus at risk of congenital defects.

Contra indications

There are no absolute contra indications to ECT. Each patient must be assessed on his merits and demerits; which carries greater risk to the patient, continuation of depressive (psychiatric) illness or a course of ECT.

ECT should not be given to a patient with raised intracranial pressure, cerebral aneurysm or a history of cerebral haemorrhage. ECT is not recommended for clients with histories of cardiovascular disease, because elevated hormone levels contribute to transient hypertension and tachycardia that may increase the risk of stroke or coronary thrombosis. It is also contraindicated for patients with a brain tumour, acute myocardial infarction, congestive heart failure, pneumonia or aortic aneurysm. Since the introduction of modified ECT there are no orthopaedic contra indications to the treatment. In particular, old age itself is not a contra indication.

Efficacy

ECT has undisputed therapeutic efficacy in melancholic depressives. It has also proven efficacy in mania as well as in schizophrenia. In comparison to antidepressants ECT is superior in depressives, and to lithium in mania. However, ECT alone is not convincingly superior to antipsychotic drugs in schizophrenia. Drugs with ECT combination, however, is superior to drug alone in schizophrenia.

Administration

ECT can be administered in a hospital, clinic or in nursing homes.

Consent

Informed consent for ECT must be obtained from patients, preferably in writing. If a patient's psychological state does not permit this, consent may be obtained from patient's legal guardian. Procedure of obtaining consent gives opportunity to educate the patient and family about ECT and allay the anxiety and fear about the treatment.

ECT team

A team consisting of psychiatrist, anaesthesiologist, trained nurses and aides should be involved in the administration of ECT.

Treatment facilities

There should be a suite of three rooms:

(i) a pleasant and comfortable waiting room (pre-ECT room)

(ii) the room where ECT is given, and

(iii) a well-equipped recovery room.

The ECT room should be equipped with (besides ECT machine and accessories) an anaesthetic appliance, suction apparatus, face masks, oxygen cylinders with adjustable flow valves, curved tongue depressors, mouth gags, resuscitation apparatus and full set of emergency drugs. There should be immediate access to a defibrillator.

122

Pre-ECT preparation

The patient receives atropine sulphate subcutaneously before the procedure to decrease oropharyngeal secretions and to block the vagus nerve so as to protect the heart from bradycardia and arryhythmias. Hitherto, atropine (1.0 mg sc/1M) was given. Now a better drug to dry up secretion is available glycopyrrolate, which does not cross the blood-brain barrier. But its usage is yet to become popular. Atropine is to be given half an hour or one hour before treatment.

Anaesthetic agents

At the beginning of ECT an intravenous dose of sodium pentothal or methohexital sodium (brevital) is given as a sedative. It is the drug of choice for ECT anaesthesia. The other drug given usually is thiopentone sodium (pentothal 5 mg/kg). After this, a muscle relaxant such as succynylcoline (1 mg/kg) is to be given. It can. be given through the same needle of pentothal but from a different syringe.

Oxygenation

This should be given through a face mask both before and after muscle relaxant induced apnoea. If this is done adequately cerebral hypoxia does not occur during ECT. The oxygen demands of the brain increases markedly during seizure; hence oxygenation is important. It also reduces the seizure threshold.

Pre-ECT preparation

Following are the nursing roles and responsibilities, which are similar to those preceeding a surgical procedure:

(i)   Check the record for recent physical examination and routine laboratory work (blood count, blood chemistries, and urine analysis). Results of pre ECT psychological evaluations of memory capacity are helpful.

(ii)   Check for a signed consent form.

(iii) Involve the family as much as possible to inform them and abate their fears and anxieties.

(iv) Communicate positive feelings about the procedure to the family and patient.

(v)   Discourage cigarette smoking just before the procedure to avoid increased difficulty in managing pulmonary secretions during treatment.

(vi) Ensure that liquids and solids are not taken six hours before treatment.

(vii) Remove dentures, glasses, jewelry, contact lens, metal hair clips, pins from the patients and dress them in loose clothing.

(viii) Have the client evacuate bladder and bowels.

(ix) Monitor vital signs before, during and after treatment.

(x)   Give atropine as ordered before treatment. It may also be given intravenously just before the treatment.

(xi) Make sure that oxygen, suction and endotracheal intubation is accessible and functional in case of a cardiorespiratory emergency.

(xii) Display a warm, supportive attitude to reduce apprehension. Patients receiving ECT are somewhat anxious (because they are familiar with the common usage of the term "shock" therapy for ECT and the word "shock" is shocking to them) especially about the first treatment. Although the procedure is painless, some feel a sense of dread since the idea of shock and subsequent seizure can be frightening.

Application of electrodes

Care must be taken in applying the electrodes. The electrodes should be suitably moistened with electrolyte jelly. The inter-electrode scalp area should be dry. The electrodes should be applied firmly throughout the passage of current. The administrator should have dry hands and all personnel should avoid direct contact with the metallic parts of the electrodes.

Electrode placement

The choice between unilateral and bilateral electrode placement is still controversial.

In bilateral ECT, electrodes are placed on each side one inch above the mid point of an imaginary line connecting the outer canthus of the eye and tragus. One of these electrode positions (right nondominant) and the other on the same side one inch lateral to vertex are used in unilateral ECT.

A mouth gag and airway are inserted, the neck extended and jaw pulled forward (to prevent the tongue from falling back and obstructing the air passages). Once the succinylcoline fasciculations have disappeared, the stimulus current is passed. Usually the stimulus will be ranging from 70 to 150 volts for a period of 0.1 to 0.5 second.

Monitoring seizure activity

It is advisable to monitor the seizure duration to ensure that the patient has experienced an adequate convulsion. Electroencephalogram (EEG) monitoring is commonly used in the West. More commonly the 'cuff' method is used to recognise and to monitor the duration of motor seizure. A blood pressure cuff (BP cuff) is placed on an arm and inflated 50 to 80 mm/mg above systolic blood pressure. This is done prior to injection of scoline in the opposite forearm. The cuffed forearm is not paralysed by scoline.

If the stimulus has failed to elicit a convulsion or if the convulsion has not been 'adequate', restimulation is permissible subject to the duration of action of the muscle relaxant. Repeated restimulations in a single treatment session, however, increase the risk of post-ECT confusion and cognitive impairment.

Re-oxygenation

The patient should be re-oxygenated after the seizure until he resumes regular and spontaneous respiration. A careful watch should be made for prolonged post-treatment apnoea.

Nurse's role during treatment

(i)   Maintain the airway and remove pharyngeal secretions with suction as necessary.

(ii) Observe the patient continuously until he is fully recovered.

(iii) Stay with the patient till he or she is fully awake.

126

After treatment

(i)   Place the patient on a side position on a railing cot.

(ii)   Touch the patient as he awakens to demonstrate care, establish your presence and allay fear.

(iii)   Orient the patient to time, place and events as he awakens.

(iv)   Give medications for minor discomforts such as headache or nausea.

(v)   Provide opportunities for the patient to express his feelings about the treatment.

(vi)   Promote normal activity after the treatment to discourage incapacity.

(vii) Give him the food as he had starved for 6 hours.

(viii) Document patient's responses during and after treatment.

(ix)   Check his vital signs and record every fifteen minutes for the first hour.

(x)   Allow him to ambulate only when he is awake, alert and able to ambulate.

Side effects

ECT is also known to produce undesirable side effects, like amnesia, confusion and EEG slowing. The post-ECT confusional state follows tonic-clonic seizures.

Memory impairment is a frequent and distressing, though for the most part reversible, consequence of ECT. It occurs in a variety of forms and its nature and severity depends to a great degree on where and how the electrical stimulus was delivered.

A variety of clinical and experimental data supports the presence of brain distabling side effects, not rarely occurring but on a permanent basis. ECT has been implicated to produce pathological, biochemical and physiological changes in the brain.

The patients complain of dizziness, dryness of moth, headache, weakness/fatigue, muscle pain, palpitation and nausea, vomiting during post-ECT period. They also present unsteady gait, poor concentration, drowsiness, anxiety, restlessness, sweating, respiratory disress, seazures (rare), tongue bite and incontinence.

Complications

Life-threatening complications of ECT are rare. Back pain occasionally results and may persists for a few days or weeks. Fractures are not uncommon in elderly patients with osteoporosis. The aged with a history of coronory disease also may develop cardiac dysrhythmia. Respiratory arrest, if it occurs, is the result of the anaesthesia or muscle relaxant.

Memory losos is a common but transient side effect. Memory for events immediately before and during the treatment remains impaired, but memory for events upto 2 years before treatment and remote memory generally returns to normal.

Although the potential for these effects appears to be minimal, the patient must be made aware of the risks involved before consenting to treatment.

Questions

1. Define ECT.

2. How does ECT act on the patient?

3. List down the indications for ECT.

4. Identify the contra indications for ECT.

5. What are the nurses role in pre-ECT period with the patients?

6. Discuss briefly the nurses role during ECT.

7. How will you take care of a patient in post ECT period?

8. What are the side effects of ECT.

9. List down the complications of ECT.

10. Write short notes on:

    i) Van Meduna

    ii) Cerletti and Bini

    iii) Types of ECT

    iv) Drugs administered prior to ECT and their purposes

    v) Electrode placement

Psychotherapy

As human beings most people experience various kinds of emotional difficulties at some time or the other in their lives. These emotional problems are frequently related to several kinds of undesirable life experiences. Problems related to family, work, education, finance, health, marriage, relationships with other people and the like are experienced by us from time to time. At times these problems may become so severe and so unbearable that unpleasant symptoms of anxiety and depression may result, interfering with normal functioning. Such problems often present in the guise of somatic complaints. Individuals experiencing such difficulties are best helped by psychotherapy rather than psychotropic medication. Treatment methods most effective in these situations involve the principles of psychotherapy and counseling. The focus of treatment is to communicate with the individual in distress, understand the source of the problem, and utilize specific psychological remedies to deal with the problems effectively.

Definition

Psychotherapy has been defined in various ways. Briefly it can be defined as "the treatment of emotional and/or related bodily problems by psychological means".

The term 'psychological means' is meant to cover a number of techniques which are mediated by verbal interaction (listening and talking). To put it another way, in psychotherapy, the helping person attempts to relieve an individual's distress by facilitating changes in his feelings, attitudes and behaviour by means of verbal and emotional communications.

Wolberg defined psychotherapy as, "the treatment by psychological means, of problems of an emotional nature, in which a trained person (therapist) deliberately establishes a professional relationship with the patient to,

(i) remove, modify or retard existing symptoms,

(ii) mediate disturbed patterns of behaviour, and/or

(iii) promote positive personality growth and development".

However, psychotherapy is the development of a trusting relationship, which allows free communication and leads to understanding, integration and acceptance of self.

Common factors of psychotherapy

In all the forms of psychotherapy, the therapist tries to help the patient to overcome emotional problems by a combination of **listening** and **talking**.

Restoration of morale is an important part of psychotherapy because most of the patients who are treated have experienced repeated failures and become demoralised, losing the conviction that they can help themselves.

Release of emotion is helpful in the early stage of treatment. Abreaction is a type of psychotherapy and it refers to a procedure in which particularly intense and rapid release of feelings is encouraged.

All forms of psychotherapy include a **rationale** that makes the patient's disorder more intelligible. This rationale may be described in detail by the therapist in behaviour therapy or short-term psychotherapy, or the patient may have to piece it together from partial explanations and interpretations as in psychoanalytically oriented psychotherapy. Rationale has the effect of making problems more understandable and therefore gives the patient more confidence that he can solve his problems.

All psychotherapy contains an element of **suggestion.** In hypnosis this is deliberately cultivated as the main agent of change.

Another component of psychotherapy is the relationship between patient and therapist. As treatment progresses, the realistic relationship or 'treatment alliance' becomes more intense, emotionally charged relationship. As a result, the patient reveals personal problems. The intimacy of the situation causes the patient to transfer to the therapist his feelings and attitudes that were originally experienced in relation to other significant persons with whom he experienced a comparable intimacy in earlier life – usually the parents. This is called as transference. When the therapist is conceived as a good figure, transference is said to be positive; when the therapist is conceived as a bad figure the transference is said to be negative.

The therapist has to remain an impartial professional and yet be genuinely concerned about the patient's most intimate problems. Despite his training, the therapist at times fail to have detachment from patient and at the same time show concern to patient's problem. Therapist may then respond in a way that is not simply a reflection of the patient's personal qualities but also a displacement on to the patient of ideas and feelings related to other figures in the therapist's life. This process is called counter-transference.

Transference and counter transference are most developed in the intensive form of treatment based on psycho-analysis, where transference is encouraged in order to use it therapeutically.

Types of psychotherapy

Psychotherapies are classified according to:

(a) Depth of probing in the unconscious mind.

   (i) Superficial or short-term (also known as supportive psychotherapy).

   (ii) Deep or long-term (also known as analytic psychotherapy).

   (iii) Educative (also known as counseling).

(b) Number of patients treated in any therapeutic session.

   (i) individual psychotherapy

   (ii) Group psychotherapy

   (iii) Family psychotherapy

(c) According to the purpose for which psychotherapy is given and the theoritical formulations used in psychotherapy.

(i)   Supportive psychotherapy : It provides support, guidance, advice and reassurance.

(ii)   Re-educative psychotherapy : It attempts to teach the individual new patterns of behaviour and social functioning.

(iii) Reconstructive psychotherapy : It aims to dismantle and rebuild a new personality.

Some commonly applied psychotherapeutic techniques

There are several types of psychotherapies. These are described below.

(i) Ventilation

Emotional problems and minor psychiatric disorders like neurosis are frequently related to several psychological and social factors. These could be in the form of various external pressures (stress factors), internal pressures (conflicts), or because of faulty learning. Often these experiences involve the subject's very personal aspects of life. As a consequence emotions get bottled up and result in a variety of symptoms. In such situations, the very process of facilitating the individual to talk about his suppressed experiences will bring down the distress. As the proverb goes 'Joy shared is doubled. Sorrow shared is halved'. This process of allowing the release of bottled up emotion is called ventilation.

Abreaction

This is a process similar to ventilation. The only difference is that the degree of emotional release is much greater here. The patient might burst out sobbing while recounting his experiences. In such circumstances, the therapist allows the person to abreact without interrupting him. The process can be facilitated by such statements as "It must have been very difficult for you" or "I understand how sad you must be feeling", etc.

(iii) Reassurance

Often we come across patients who have marked anxiety over their symptoms. For example, a person experiencing chest pain may fear that it is indicative of a serious physical illness. Similarly, many other patients express doubts as to whether they would get well at all. In such situations it is necessary to alleviate the person's anxiety with reassuring statements like, "you do not have a serious problem. I am confident that you will get well".

(iv) Explanation

Patients and family members may often have an inadequate understanding of the nature and cause of the illness resulting in anxiety about the illness. Explanations should be provided to remove misconceptions and to provide a proper understanding of the problem.

(v) Suggestion

Suggestion is a process by which symptoms relief is achieved through positive statements made with a degree of firmness and authority. Suggestion often works well when the subject displays a high degree of faith in the therapist. Examples of suggestive statements are:

"You will feel confident henceforth"

"You will not experience headache any more"

Suggestion is always beneficial in neurotics and psychosomatic conditions.

However, suggestion must be employed along with other techniques. For example, suggestion might help the removal of a hysterical symptom. But further exploration may be necessary to understand the cause of the hysterical symptom. Based on the cause of the problem, more specific treatment needs to be instituted.

(vi) Persuasion

Persuasion is a procedure by which the therapist urges the patient repeatedly to change his behaviour or to try new methods of dealing with his problem.

(vii) Reinforcement

Reinforcements or rewards are potent methods to enhance the desired behaviour. They can be verbal or material in nature. Verbal reinforcers include statements like "you have done well", "excellent", "I am happy that you have begun to work", etc. Such statements should be associated with the appropriate gestures. Material reinforcers are often used in children. For example, eatables or play materials can be given immediately after the child shows desirable behaviour.

(viii) Recreation

Recreation helps to break monotony of work. It is especially required for subjects who have developed emotional problems as a result of having to perform monotonous and hard work. The therapist suggests such activities as listening to radio, going for a movie/drama, playing indoor games, attending bhajans, playing with children or going out for a refreshing walk.

(ix) Work as therapy

Work is an important form of therapy for many types of emotional problems. When a person engages in work, his preoccupation with his problems get lessened. It enhances his self-esteem since he is not dependent on others. Sometimes work can even be a healthy way of resolving conflict.

(x) Relaxation

Relaxation is a technique especially useful for anxious individuals. When a person is tense, his muscles are in a state of contraction, and this produces muscular pains. By voluntary effort the individual can learn to relax his muscles and experience relief from tension pains. Relaxation is also beneficial for a variety of psychosomatic problems like hypertension, peptic ulcer/hyperacidity, bronchial asthma, and migraine.

Techniques like Shavasana and Yogasana (Yoga) have also been proved to be beneficial to reduce mental tension and restore physical health.

Unwanted effects of psychotherapy

(i)   Patients may become excessively dependent on therapy or therapist.

(ii) Intensive psychotherapy may be distressing to the patient and result in exacerbation of symptoms and deterioration in relationships.

(iii) Disorders for which physical treatments would be more appropriate may be missed.

(iv) Ineffective psychotherapy wastes time and money, and damages patient's morale.

Contra indications

(i) Psychotic patients with severe behaviour disturbances like excitement.

(ii) Organic psychosis (in acute phase)

(iii) Patients who are unmotivated and unwilling sto accept it.

(iv) Group psychotherapy in hysteria, hypochondriasis, etc.

(v) Patients who are unlikely to respond, e.g. personality disorders (especially antisocial type), malingering, etc.

The phases of psychotherapy is detailed in the next topic under psychoanalytically oriented psychotherapy.

Questions

1. Define psychotherapy.

2. Discuss the types of psychotherapy.

3. Enumerate the psychotherapeutic techniques that are commonly applied.

4. Name the contra indications for psychotherapy.

5. List down the unwanted effects of psychotherapy.

6. What are the factors influence psychotherapy?

7. Write short notes on:

   i) Ventilation

   ii) Abreaction

   iii) Reinforcement

   iv) Reassurance

   v) Relaxation

Hypnosis

Hypnosis is considered to be an adjunct to psychotherapy. Nothing can be done in psychotherapy with hypnosis that cannot also be done without hypnosis. The advantage of hypnosis lies in the fact that it serves to accelerate, sometimes considerably, the impact of psychotherapeutic interventions.

The derivation of the word "hypnosis" – from the Greek word hypnos, meaning sleep – can be misleading because the phenomenon to which it refers is not a form of sleep; rather, it is a complex process of heightened or aroused concentration. Although peripheral awareness is reduced in sleep and hypnosis alike, focal awareness, which is almost obliterated in sleep, is at optimal capacity in hypnosis.

Hypnotic phenomena were first mentioned as a therapeutic tool in the 18th century by Mesmer, who refer to hypnosis as "animal magnetism". In the next century, Braid, Charcot, Liebeault, Bernheim, Janet, Freud and many others studied hypnotic phenomena.

Definition

Hypnosis can be described as an altered state of intense and sensitive interpersonal relatedness between hypnotist and patient, characterised by the state of attentive, receptive, concentration with a relative suspension of peripheral awareness.

Hypnosis can be induced in many ways. The main requirements are that the subject should be willing to be hypnotized and convinced that hypnosis will occur. Most procedures contain some combination of the following elements: relaxation and slowed respiration, a fixed point for attention (such as a moving object), rhythmic monotonous instructions, and the use of a graduated series of suggestions, (for example, that the arm will rise from the patient's side). The therapist uses the suggestible state either to implant direct suggestions of improvement or to encourage recall of previously repressed memories.

Technique

Patient is either made to lie down on a bed or sit in a chair. The patient is asked to gaze fixedly on a ring or a coin, or a spot on the wall or ceiling while the therapist makes monotonous suggestions of relaxation and sleep. He tells the patient that his eyes are getting more tired, that he is feeling drowsier, that the eyes are closing and that he is getting sleepy. This suggestion goes on till the patient's eyes flicker, lower and close and breathing takes on the characteristics of a sleeping rhythm. The patient, however, is not asleep and can hear what is being said, answer questions and obey instructions.

Indications

In psychiatry, hypnosis can be used in several ways. The first and simplest use, which requires only a light trance, is as a form of relaxation. This is used to get better control over their actions. The second use, which requires a deeper trance, is to enhance reception of suggestion in order to relieve symptoms, especially those of hysteria. Although this procedure is often effective, at least in the short term, it has not been proved better than more gradual forms of suggestion with no trance. Moreover, the sudden removal of symptoms by hypnosis is sometimes followed by an intense emotional reaction of anxiety or depression. The third use of hypnosis is an aid to psychotherapy, by bringing about the recall of repressed memories; but there is no evidence that this improves the effects of treatment.

Hypnosis is used otherwise for the following conditions :

(i) Psycho-somatic disorder, e.g., asthma, eczema, peptic ulcer, ulcerative colitis.

(ii) Tics and habitual spasms, including stammering.

(iii) Anaesthesia (in patients who are apprehensive of anaesthetic agents or cases in which it is contra indicated).

(iv) Pregnancy and labour (to induce anaesthesia and for relaxation).

(v) Hypnotherapy (to recover lost memories).

(vi) Children's functional disorders, e.g., stammering, tics, nocturnal enuresis and phobias.

(vii) Psycho-dermatological problems, e.g., warts, psoriasis, urticaria.

(viii) Other psychiatric disorders, e.g., anxiety neurosis, phobias, insomnia, pain syndromes.

Factors involved in hypnosis

Hypnotic experience involves the following three factors:

(i) Absorption

Hypnotized individuals are intensely absorbed in their trance experience.

(ii) Dissociation

The intense absorption means that many routine experiences that would ordinarily be conscious occur out of ordinary conscious awareness. Such experiences can be both induced and reversed with the structural use of hypnosis.

(iii) Suggestibility

While hypnotized individuals are not deprived of their will, they do have a tendency to accept uncritical instructions in trance, suspending the usual conscious editing functions.

Effects of hypnosis

In the somnambulistic state, suggestions can be made which can influence the patient's mental or physical state such as easing of breathing in asthmatics. Anaesthesia can be suggested and this can be localised to one limb or one eye, memories can be reactivated, regression can be induced and the patient brought back to experience again events in his earlier life which had been repressed. Hallucinatory experiences may be induced.

143

Post-hypnotic effects

After the subject has been brought out of the somnambulistic state, suggestions which were given during it can still operate and is exploited in treatment.

Contra indications

(i) Hysterical personality

The patients with hysterical character may go into so called irreversible hypnotic states, false accusations against the hypnotist, litigation and other difficulties.

(ii) Schizophrenia

Pseudoneurotic types of cases especially with their somatic preoccupations may be mistaken for anxiety or conversion disorder and may precipitate psychosis.

(iii) Paranoid states

(iv) Psychotic depression

(v) Obsessional states

Psycho-therapeutic application of hypnosis

Aim to solve the patient's problem. Hypnosis enables the psychiatrist to focus the patient's intense concentration on certain areas. The desired information can be reached more directly though hypnosis than when the psychiatrist must depend on the patient's free association with its mass resistances, irrelevant information and conscious censure. Since the patient's intensified transference and attention are focused on the treatment situation, an atmosphere of receptivity enhances his capacity for exploration and change.

Success of hypnosis mainly relies on the psychiatrist's ability to hypnotise a patient, and also his knowledge and skills in helping the patient to move forward relevant therapeutic goals.

Advantages

The adjunctive role of hypnosis lies in its ability to reduce the time needed for treatment by cutting through the patient's resistance, thereby permitting the therapist to use transference as a therapeutic device, operative in a desirable direction. The effectiveness of hypnosis depends on the patient's well-being and it is determined by the following conditions:

(i)   restoration of the patient's previous level of self-esteem;

(ii)   the alleviation of stress in his environment;

(iii) the patient's reformulation of the symbolism of his symptom into a less extreme form;

(iv)   the provision of clinical atmosphere to re orient himself in strengthening his self-respect.

The use of hypnosis to facilitate psychotherapy involves two basic strategies: the first strategy is to enhance the patient's control; the second is to uncover the material the patient has repressed. And the same may be used during different phases of psychotherapy.

Control enhancement : This mode of hypnosis is usually focused upon (i) symptom alteration or (ii) attitude alteration, as substitutive and diversionary

145

experiences. These are essentially suppressive and containment operations, designed to increase the patient's control so that he can learn more effective ways of achieving the defined goals of his thΛrapy.

Symptom alteration is simply a direct guidance which keeps the patient's attention away from his symptoms and concomitantly reminds him that more resourceful and effective means are available for his use in coping with problems of adaptation. For example, an embarassing exposed head tic may be converted to a hidden toe tic and the phobic reactor can learn to differentiate real danger from generalised fear, and a confused, disoriented person can re-establish time, place and self-identity.

Attitude alteration : Presents the patient with an alternative attitude towards a chronic, recurrent disability or a pending problematic event; and, by invoking the power of compulsive compliance, patient's adaptation efficiency increased. For example, compulsive cigarette smoking can be stopped when the patient concentrates on his new need to respect his body and to protect it from poison; pain can be endured when a mother wants to experience the birth process and to deliver her baby without chemical anaesthesia; phonation can return when the aphonic patient learns a new way to express and cope with a secret, critical grievance; psychogenic paralysis can be cured when the patient realises that he no longer has the need for invalidism.

Uncovering repressed material : Uncovering which is repressed that (both affective and cognitive content), may be accomplished (i) by simple abreaction or (ii) by more complex exploration of past events.

146

(i) Abreaction

The release of repressed material can sometimes be provoked by design. It is employed usually in patients whose syndromes developed as a result of recent situational catastrophic experiences – such as war, fire or accident – which, if not uncovered, may develop into traumatic neuroses.

(ii) Explorative uncovering

This is the most subtle form of hypnotic intervention in psychotherapy. It makes use of the hyperamnesia that is possible in this state of aroused concentration and it is a valuable data collecting procedure, especially when amnesia for specific events is at issue.

Precautions

In general, hypnosis is remarkably safe when it is used with sound clinical judgement, in a goal directed setting. In a broader sense, the use of hypnosis as an uncovering device demands certain precautions and should be performed only by those clinicians who are adequately trained in reconstructive psychotherapeutic techniques.

When a therapist commits an error while the patient is in trance state, it becomes ready access for the patient to adopt to the error than critically judging. Therefore, hypnosis is reserved for those clinicians who have been trained in the psychodynamics of intervention.

Questions

1. Define hypnosis.

2. Discuss the techniques used to induce hypnosis.

3. Name the indications for hypnosis.

4. What are the factors influence hypnosis?

5. How does hypnosis affect an individual?

6. List down the contra indications for hypnosis.

7. How do you explain the psychotherapeutic application of hypnosis?

8. What are the advantages of hypnosis?

9. How does hypnosis facilitate psycho therapy?

10. Explain the strategy of control enhancement through hypnosis.

11. What are the techniques used for uncovering repressed material through hypnosis?

12. What precautions do you need to keep in mind before suggesting for hypnosis to a patient?

Psychoanalysis

Psychoanalysis is the most time-consuming form of psychotherapy. Its practitioners receive lengthy training which involves personal analysis as well as supervised experience in treating patients. For these reasons and because results have not been shown to be better than those of shorter forms of treatment, psychoanalysis is not widely used in our country.

Definition

Psychoanalysis is a procedure for the investigation of unconscious psychical processes, otherwise inaccessible. It is also a therapeutic technique of treating psychiatric disorders by psychological means.

Basic concepts about psychoanalysis

The credit for the 'invention' of psychoanalysis belongs to Sigmund Freud (1856-1939).

Topographic theory of mind

This theory was advanced in the year 1900 in "the interpretation of dreams". Although it was later almost replaced by the structural theory, it is still useful in understanding the mental mechanisms.

The three divisions of mind according to this theory, are the unconscious, the pre-conscious and the conscious.

(i) The unconscious : Much of the mental activity lies outside the sphere of consciousness. Still, it influences the conscious thought and behaviour even if it is not available to voluntary recall.

The unconscious contains those ideas and affects which have been repressed (by "the censor", as the repression mechanism is known). These repressed materials can only reach the consciousness through the preconscious when the censor is relaxed and free from threat to security (e.g. dreams, abreaction), or is over powered (e.g. tongue slips, free association).

(ii) The pre-conscious : This region of mind lies between the unconscious and the conscious with access to both. The unconscious mental contents can reach the conscious only through the pre-conscious. The censor lies here maintaining the repressive barrier.

The pre-conscious mental contents can easily become conscious with the focusing of attention.

(iii) The conscious : The conscious constitutes a tiny position of the mind. Freud conceptualised it as a type of special sense organ of attention concerned with registration of stimuli from both within and without.

From the Iceberg theory, the three levels of mind could be explained as follows. When the ice piece is floating in water, some part of ice is exposed and that is the conscious; the portion of ice piece just underneath the water level is the "pre-conscious; and the remaining part of ice piece which is totally submerged is called the unconscious.

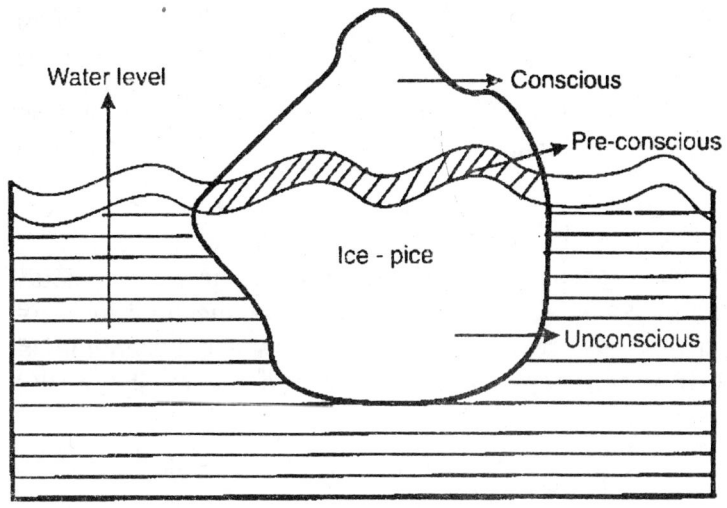

Water level

Conscious

Pre-conscious

Ice - pice

Unconscious

Iceberg theory to explain division of mind

In addition to the topographic model of mind, Freud also theorised the concept of psychic determinism which means that all mental activity is meaningful and purposeful, though unconscious, and is linked with previous life experiences. Hence no mental activity can be accidental or purposeless.

Structural theory of mind

In 1923, Freud divided the mental apparatus into three dynamic structures: the id, the ego and the superego.

(i) **The id :** It is the original state of human mental apparatus with which a baby is born. It is totally unconscious, containing the basic drives and instincts

151

concerned with survival, sexual drive and aggression. It is characterised by primary process thinking and is based on pleasure seeking principle, lacking any direct link with reality. The only urge of these drives is immediate gratification.

(ii) The ego : The ego is primarily determined by the experience of reality and is therefore guided by the reality seeking principle. It is predominantly conscious, though some parts (like ego defense mechanisms) are unconscious. Ego maintains a balance between the id and the superego on one hand and the reality on the other.

The ego is the seat of conscious, intellectual, self-preservative and defensive functions of mental apparatus.

(iii) The superego : The superego is a pre-dominantly unconscious subdivision of mental apparatus that develops from the ego. It is specially concerned with moral standards (morality seeking principle) and has two parts – a punitive conscience and a nonpunitive ego idea. Both derive from the effect of parental influence on the ego. This parental influence not only includes the effect of actual parents but also of other important family members, religion and important people in the surrounding environment.

The mechanism of ego defense

The term "ego defense mechanism" refers to the various automatic, involuntary and unconsciously instituted psychological activities by which the unacceptable urges or impulses are excluded from conscious awareness. These defense mechanisms are a function of the ego.

The defense mechanisms usually operate on an unconscious level (except suppression, which is a voluntary defense mechanism). In contrast, coping mechanisms are voluntary and conscious mechanisms of defense which an individual employs to deal with day-to-day external and conscious fears and conflicts.

No ego defense mechanism is psychotic, neurotic, immature, mature or normal. All mechanisms of defense are used by normal individuals. It is an exclusive or abnormally excessive use that makes a defense mechanism neurotic or psychotic.

4. The theory of psycho-sexual development

In 1905, Freud described the psycho-sexual stages of development. They are:

(i) Oral phase (Birth to 1 - 1½ years): Infant gets gratification through the oral region.

Fixation at and regression to this stage leads to dependent personality traits, schizophrenia, severe mood disorder, alcohol dependence syndrome and drug dependence behaviour.

(ii) Anal phase (1 - 1½ years to 3 years): Child gets gratification through the anal and peri-anal area. Ma; r achievement is toilet training (sphincter control).

Fixation at this stage leads to obsessive-compulsive personality traits and obsessive-compulsive disorder.

(iii) Phallic phase (3 to 5 years) or oedipal phase: Major site of gratification is the genital area.

Fixation at this stage leads to sexual deviations, sexual dysfunctions and neurotic disorders.

(iv) Latency phase (5 to 6 years to 12 years): This is a stage of relative sexual quiescence. Super ego is formed at this stage. Sexual drive is channelised into socially appropriate goals like development of interpersonal relationships, sports, school work, etc.

Fixation at this stage leads to neurotic disorders.

(v) Genital phase (12 years onwards/puberty onwards): Adult sexuality develops with capacity for intimacy and respect for others. Gradual release from parental controls with more influence of peer group is seen.

Fixation at this stage leads to neurotic disorders.

5. Theory of dreams

Dream interpretation is a major component of psychoanalysis. Beginning with his dream experiences, Freud analysed dreams as "the royal road to the unconscious". He believed dreams to be conscious expression of unconscious fantasies or impulses which are not accessible to the individual in wakefulness, thereby providing gratification by wish fulfillment.

Since expression of unconscious, forbidden fantasies can evoke considerable anxiety, these fantasies are considerably modified so as to preserve sleep on the one hand and provide gratification of the fantasies on the other. This modification is known as dream work. Here the unconscious, forbidden fantasies or wishes which threaten to break sleep constitute the latent dream content, whereas the dream content modified by dream work constitutes the manifest dream content. According to Freud, the aim of dream interpretation is to get to the latent dream content from manifest dream content via free association, in order to understand the "real meaning" of the dream experience.

The dream work consists of the following mechanisms :

(i)   Symbolism

(ii)   Displacement

(iii)   Condensation

(iv)   Projection

(v)   Secondary elaboration (since dream content consists of primary process thinking, sec-ondary elaboration is used to introduce logical thinking or secondary process thinking in the dream content).

I   **Classical psychoanalysis : (Freudian)**

A detailed discussion of Freudian psychoanalysis is not attempted here. A very brief outline of the therapy is presented.

It needs 3-5 visits/week by the patient for a period of 3-5 years (even longer). No history taking, examination or diagnosis is attempted. Patient is allowed to communicate unguided by 'free association'. (Free association is the spontaneous, uncensored verbalisation by the patient of whatever comes to mind).

The therapist remains passive and his approach is non-directive. He constantly challenges existing

155

'defenses' and interprets 'resistence'. (Interpretation is the process by which the therapist brings the patient to an understanding of a particular aspect of his problems or behaviour. The resistence is patient's conscious or unconscious psychologic defense against bringing repressed/ unconscious thoughts to light).

Transference and counter transference takes place during therapy. No advice is ever given to the patient. The crux of the therapy is on interpretation.

During the therapy, the patient typically lies on the couch, with the therapist just out of vision.

II Psychoanalytically oriented psychotherapy

It is a much more direct form of psychoanalysis. The duration of therapy is much briefer and advice is given to the patient occasionally. The patient and the therapist sit face to face. Additional modes of treatment including drug therapy can be used.

Indications

(i)   Presence of long-standing mental conflicts which, although are unconscious, produce symptomatology.

(ii) High motivation to undergo therapy.

(iii) Patient should have strong 'ego-structure' which can bear frustrations of impulses during therapy.

(iv) Patient should be psychologically minded and should not have significant life stressors.

(v)   Neurotic disorder, personality disorder.

Phases

Usually the therapy proceeds through three broad phases, namely: an initial phase, a middle phase, and a terminal phase. These phases are not rigidly delineated and the progress from one phase to another will vary from patient to patient. However, certain major themes can be identified in each of these phases.

(i) The initial phase

The focus of this phase of therapy is to get a clear understanding of the nature and cause of the patient's problem and to provide an explanation of the nature of therapy. This phase usually lasts two to four sessions and includes the following steps.

(a) **Evaluation of the patient** : A detailed evaluation is a prerequisite before beginning therapy. It is done by collecting detail history from the patient, from the family members or friends, doing physical and mental state examinations.

(b) **Explanation of the nature of treatment** : It is not uncommon for patients to view their problems as medical conditions even though they suffer from a primary emotional disturbance. As a result they expect to be treated by medicines. They do not readily accept the possibility of resolving their difficulties by talking with the therapist. Hence it is necessary that the therapist explains in detail the psychotherapeutic intervention that is being recommended as the main treatment.

(c) **Development of an empathic relationship** : The therapist should attempt to build a trusting

157

relationship with the patient to enable the patient to share his difficulties. Empathy is the process by which the therapist attempts to understand the emotional state of the patient by trying to place himself in the patient's situation. This is in contrast to sympathy where the depth of emotional involvement is lesser. Often the very process of empathic understanding greatly relieves the patient's distress.

(d) **Exploration of the problems and stress factors:** The therapist should initiate attempts to understand the specific stress factors or conflicts which have been responsible for the patient's emotional difficulties. This is frequently a slow process and may extend on to the next phase of therapy.

(ii) **The middle phase**

This phase which usually takes about three to five sessions focuses on the problems and the application of specific therapeutic techniques to deal with these problems.

(a) **Strengthening of the therapeutic relationship :** As the patient and therapist continue to interact, the therapeutic relationship becomes stronger. The individual becomes more open to understand the source of his problems and try different methods of dealing with his difficulties.

(b) **Further understanding of the patient's life situation :** By a process of listening to the life history of the patient, the therapist gets a fuller understanding of the patient's problems. During this phase, some individuals may continue to experience anxiety about discussing their problems because of the fear that the therapist may disapprove them. In the interaction, this 'resistance' manifests itself in the form of long pauses, silences or diverting the topic. The therapist should handle such blocks by gently reassuring the patient and conveying his positive regard irrespective of what the patient reveals.

(c) **Application of therapeutic techniques** : The therapist uses a number of techniques to alleviate the patient's emotional distress. Some of these techniques are ventilation, abreaction, suggestion, persuation, reinforcement, reassurance and explanation. (These are described earlier under the topic 'psychotherapy').

(d) **Enabling the development of insight** : Insight refers to the understanding by the patient, of the origin and nature of his problems. Through the use of the above mentioned techniques, the therapist enables the development of insight. The patient becomes aware of causal link between the conflicts/ stress factors and the symptoms.

(iii) **The end phase**

The next 3-4 sessions constitute the terminal phase. It includes :

(a) **Strengthening of insight :** Patient's understanding of the problem is strengthened by restating the silent themes that emerge during therapy.

(b) **Reinforcing the patient's improvement** : As the therapy continues, the patient learns new methods of dealing with his difficulties, and simultaneously his symptoms reduce. The therapist should positively reinforce the patient's improvement through assurances such as, "I am happy to note that you are able to deal with your problems better now. If you continue to work along the same lines, I am sure you will be fully capable of managing by yourself".

(c) **Preparing the patient for termination of treatment:** This is done in a gradual fashion. The therapy sessions are spaced out, thus paving way for a formal termination. Sometimes patients might resist termination of therapy because of the belief that the therapist will be ever present to solve all their problems. This is called dependence. The therapist must undo this dependence by gently bringing it to the patient's notice.

The frequency of patient meeting psychotherapist once a week is sufficient. But in crisis situations like suicidal threats, it may be preferable to see the patient more frequently, i.e., once in two or three days. Once the patient has shown satisfactory improvement, it is sufficient to see the patient once in a month.

The length of sessions ranges from few minutes to 30 minutes. But this can be adjusted by the therapist based on his working pattern and the needs of the patient.

The number of such sessions may be between 5-10 as required for most of the patients. However, improvement may be seen earlier or later than this.

Questions

1. Define psychoanalysis.

2. What are the basic concepts involved in psycho-analysis.

3. Explain the structural theory of mind.

4. How does defense mechanisms operate?

5. Discuss the theory of psycho-sexual development.

6. How does Sigmond Freud used 'dreams' in psychoanalysis?

7. What are the salient features of classical psychoanalysis?

8. List down the indications for psycho-analysis.

9. How do you conduct psycho-analytically oriented psychotherapy?

10. Write short notes on :

   i) Sigmond Freud

   ii) Id

   iii) Ego

   iv) Super ego

   iv) Phases of psycho-sexual development of an individual

   v) Empathy

   ━━━━━━━━━━

Behaviour therapy

The term behaviour therapy is applied to psychological treatments based on experimental psychology and intended to change symptoms and behaviour. Two other terms are used to describe these methods: behaviour modification, is employed both as a synonym for behaviour therapy and to refer to a particular group of procedures based on operant conditioning; behavioural psychotherapy generally refers to behaviour therapies other than operant methods. The term cognitive therapy is applied to psychological treatment intended to change maladaptive ways of thinking and thereby bring about improvement in psychiatric disorders.

Definition

Broadly defined, behaviour therapy is a type of psychotherapy which is based on theories of learning, and aims at changing maladaptive behaviour and substituting it with adaptive behaviour.

Theories of learning

Although, there are many theories of learning, a majority of behaviour therapy techniques are based on operant conditioning model (Skinner, 1953) and classical conditioning model (Pavlov, 1849-1936).

162

Classical conditioning (CC)

Ivan P. Pavlov demonstrated the essential operation in classical conditioning (CC) is a pairing of two stimuli.

A neutral conditioned stimulus (CS) is paired with an unconditioned stimulus (US) that evokes an unconditioned response (UR). As a result of this pairing, the previously neutral conditioned stimulus begins to call forth a response similar to that evoked by the unconditioned stimulus. After learning, when the conditioned stimulus produces the response, the response is called a conditioned response (CR).

Operant conditioning (OC)

B. F. Skinner demonstrated, using a reinforcer, that operant conditioning (OC), is any stimulus or event which, when produced by a response, makes that response more likely to occur in future.

The major principle of OC is that if a reinforcement is contingent upon a certain response, that response will become more likely to occur.

Techniques

(i) Systematic desensitization

This is based on reciprocal inhibition (Wolpe, 1958) principle. If a response incompatible with anxiety is made to occur at the same time as an anxiety provoking stimulus, then anxiety is reduced by reciprocal inhibition.

Systematic desensitization as given by Wolpe involves the following three stages :

(a) Training the patient to relax.

(b) Hierarchy construction, i.e., constructing with the patient a hierarchy of anxiety-arousing situation. Here the patient is asked to list all the conditions which provoke anxiety. Then he is asked to list them in a descending order of anxiety provocation. Thus a heirarchy of anxiety-producing stimuli is prepared.

(c) Systematic desensitization proper : This can be done either in imagery (SD-I) or in reality in-vivo (SD-R). At first, the lowest item in heirarchy is confronted (in reality or in imagery). Patient is advised to signal whenever anxiety is produced. With each signal, he is asked to relax (step-1). After a few trials, patient is able to control his anxiety.

Thus, gradually the heirarchy is climbed till the maximum anxiety-provoking stimulus can be faced in absence of anxiety.

This is a treatment of choice in phobias and obsessive-compulsive disorders.

(ii) Flooding

Flooding involves exposing patients to a phobic object or situation in a non-graded manner with no attempt to reduce anxiety. Unlike systematic desensitization, no prior relaxation techniques are taught to the patient, and it is usually given in a non-graded manner or in reverse heirarchy (starting from most phobic to least phobic stimulus). It can be conducted in imagination (implosion) or in vivo.

164

This is a method used in the treatment of phobias. Here the person is directly exposed to the phobic stimulus, but escape is made impossible. By prolonged contact with the phobic stimulus, therapist's guidance and encouragement and therapist's modeling behaviour, anxiety decreases.

(iii) Aversion therapy

It involves producing an unpleasant sensation in the patient, usually by influencing pain in association with a stimulus.

This is used for the treatment of those conditions which are pleasant but undesirable, e.g., alcohol dependence and transvestism, homosexuality and other sexual deviations.

The underlying principle is the pairing of the pleasant stimulus (e.g. alcohol) with an unpleasant response, so that even in absence of the unpleasant response (after therapy is over), the pleasant stimulus becomes unpleasant by association.

The unpleasant aversion is produced by electric stimulus (low voltage), drugs (like apomorphine and disulfiram) or even by fantasy (when it is called covert sensitization).

Typically, 20-40 sessions are given, with each session lasting about 1 hour. After completion of treatment, booster sessions may be given.

(iv) Operant conditioning procedures for increasing a behaviour

(a) Positive reinforcement The desirable behaviour is reinforced by a reward, material or symbolic.

(b)   Negative reinforcement : On performance of the desirable behaviour, punishment can be avoided.

(c)   Modeling : The person is exposed to a 'model' behaviour and is induced to copy it. This can be used to avoid certain behaviours.

(v)   Operant conditioning procedures for decreasing a behaviour

(a)   Time-out : Here, the reinforcement is withdrawn for some time, contingent upon the undesired response. This is often used in therapy with children. For example, the child is not allowed to go out of the ward to play when he fails to complete the given work.

(b)   Punishment : Aversive stimulus is here presented, contingent upon the undesirable response. That is, whenever the undesired response occurs, punishment is given.

(c)   Satiation : The undesired response is positively reinforced, so that tiring occurs. A similar technique is negative practice procedure.

(vi)   Negative practice (Dunlap, 1932)

Some problems, e.g., tics, stammering, thumbsucking, nail biting, etc. can be reduced when the patient deliberately repeats the behaviour.

(vii)   Relaxation training

The simplest behavioural treatment for generalised anxiety disorders is relaxation training. Jacobson (1938) originally described progressive relaxation, an elaborate procedure intended to bring about reduction of tonus in individual groups of skeletal muscles and to regulate breathing.

(viii) Assertiveness training

Assertiveness training is designed to encourage direct but socially acceptable expression of thoughts and feelings by people who are shy or socially awkward. The method was first described by Salter (1949) and developed by Wolpe (1958). The essence of the treatment is that patients enact social encounters in which a degree of self-assertion would be appropriate; for example, being ignored by a gossiping shop assistant. By a combination of coaching, modeling, and role-reversal patients are encouraged to practice appropriate verbal and non-verbal behaviour.

Indications

Behaviour therapy is a treatment of choice in:

Phobias

Compulsions

Nocturnal enuresis

Social anxiety states

Sexual dysfunction

Tension headaches

Tics

Obesity

Anorexia nervosa

Also used to modify:

Maladaptive habits

Sexual role disturbances

Psychosomatic reactions

Smoking

Drinking

Contra indications

Those psychiatric disorders in which symptomatology is acute, pervasive or non-circumscribed and in which triggering environmental events or external reinforcement are not obvious or capable of definition.

Questions

1. Define behaviour therapy.
2. What is classical conditioning?
3. How do you explain operant conditioning?
4. Discuss briefly the techniques used in behaviour therapy.
5. What are the indications and contra indications for behaviour therapy?
6. Write short notes on :
   i)   Systematic desensitization
   ii)   Flooding
   iii) Aversion therapy
   iv)   Relaxation training in behaviour therapy
   v)   Assertiveness training

Recreational and social therapy

Recreational Therapy

Recreation is a form of activity therapy used in most psychiatric settings. Therapeutic recreation can occur as informal ping-pong and card games, structured soft ball, basket ball or volley ball games, as trips outside the hospital, attending sports events, and so on. Recreation or play activities provide patients with the opportunity for fun and for feeling good. It tends balance to their daily schedule and helps in treating the whole patient.

Play is one kind of recreational therapy. It is considered as a variety of occupations that constitute a pleasurable way of passing time and are also the medium through which a wide range of skills can be learned and rehearsed.

Nurses can use a recreational activity as a foothold for establishing a therapeutic relationship with patients or as a platform for therapeutic encounters with patients who are frightened, withdrawn or reluctant to participate. Some patients view games as being non-threatening and are able to tolerate informal interactions during a game of pool, ping-pong or soft ball. Patients who play games with each other experience predictability, security, order and success they can see and feel and acceptance by a group. Nurses can be role models of healthy behaviours for patients if they can display a sense of humor while engaging in therapeutic recreation. The familiar axiom of "laughter is the best medicine" helps patients discharge tension and anxiety. A structured exercise group can also help relieve tension. It can be scheduled in the morning to help patients feel better physically as they start their day and to give them a sense of accomplishment and participation. It is beneficial for hyperactive patients because it channels their energy constructively within a specific framework.

The theory of recreational therapy holds that the relationship of one's physical self to the immediate environment is important to the individual's total health. Recreational therapy provides them useful leisure activities and help them develop skills in engaging in healthy, competitive interactions.

The chief emphasis of recreational therapy is on the social re-education of the patient, and the basic objective may be described as the restoration of some function, e.g., power of attention, previously learned but for the time being inhibited or temporarily lost because of some personality change due to mental illness. Re-education is a replacement of bad habits by better habits, or the formation of new habits to replace habits which have been lost. The principle of "learning by doing" is more used in recreational therapy.

Classification of recreational activities

The various forms of play or activity used in recreational therapy are:

(i) Motor forms : These can be further divided into fundamental and accessory, based on whether the motor element is the main purpose of the

170

activity or merely incidental to it. Among the fundamental forms are such games as hockey and football, while the accessory forms are exemplified by play-activity and dancing.

(ii) The sensory forms may be either visual, e.g., looking at motion pictures, play, etc., or auditory, such as listening to a concert.

(iii) The intellectual forms include such activities as reading, debating, etc.

In recreational therapy recreation is regarded in its every sphere, and the following shows the wide range in which it is used :

(a) Goal games, e.g., hide and seek

(b) Team games, e.g., hockey and football

(c) Country sports, e.g., shooting, fishing

(d) Combats, e.g., wrestling, boxing

(e) Curiosity play, e.g., crossword puzzles

(f) Creative play, e.g., play-acting

(g) Vicarious play, e.g., viewing at motion pictures

(h) Imitative play, e.g., follow the leader in folk dancing

(i) Social play, e.g., party games

(j) Aesthetic play, e.g., painting and clay modeling

(k) Acquisition play, e.g., collecting antiques or stamps

2. Aims of recreational therapy

(i) to train memory and concentration

(ii) to re-educate mentally, physically and socially

(iii) to give a sense of responsibility, e.g., by giving an opportunity to organise or lead a game

(iv) to stimulate interest

(v) to stimulate or recreate self-confidence

(vi) to arouse and develop attention

(vii) to give an opportunity for self-expression

(viii) to replace unhealthy trends by healthy ones

(ix) to substitute encouragement for discouragement

(x) to improve the appetite

(xi) to improve the circulation

(xii) to improve respiration

(xiii) to strengthen the tone of the muscles

(xiv) to develop a sense of rhythm

(xv) to develop a good posture

Recreational therapy may also use community resources to help patients identify socialisation activities that they can become involved with after discharge from the hospital. Movement or dance therapy is a specific example of how the body can be used as a medium for change. Since body and mind cannot be separated, through dance, nurses work toward integrating the muscular and cognitive expressions of the patient's feelings and thoughts.

172

Social therapy

Social therapy is an attempt to help people to change by affecting the way in which they live. It is also a way of 'using social and organisational means to produce desired changes in people. Social therapy is about personal change and growth and living-learning experience.

The aim of social therapy is to enhance patients' activity, freedom, and responsibility. This is achieved by granting as much responsibility and freedom of action as possible to each of the several participants in the entire therapeutic team.

Social therapy in psychiatry is about two centuries old; before the eighteenth century there were hardly any institutions for the mentally ill. At the end of the eighteenth century, the 'humane revolution in psychiatry', institutional psychiatry began to develop and social therapy began.

The system of social therapy is known as moral management and it might be defined as organised group-living in which the integration and continuity of work, play and social activities produce a meaningful total life experience in which the growth of individual capacity to enjoy life has maximum opportunity.

The most important development in social therapy in the last twenty years has been the therapeutic community and it is the first to apply social therapy as the primary therapeutic process. The immediate aim of this is a full participation of all its members in its daily life and the eventual aim of resocialisation of the neurotic individual for life in ordinary society (T. Main, 1946).

The distinctive aspect of therapeutic community is 'the way the institution's total resources, both staff and patients, are self-consciously pooled in furthering treatment'. The morning meeting is where all the members of the community analyse the matters of general interest. There is a system of feedback of the events of the previous twenty-four hours. This is followed always by a staff review session, where the main meeting is analysed and personal contributions and reactions assessed. It also includes workshop groups, domestic groups, small psychotherapy groups, staff sensitivity groups, assessment sessions, etc. In all these there is some immediate business, but the main task is the social analysis of the 'here and now' – what is happening amongst the members of the groups at that time – always with the eventual aim of increasing the individual's awareness and understanding of what he is doing to himself and to other people.

1. Importance of social therapy

When the patients admitted into mental hospital, they tend to develop "Institutional Neurosis". It is a disease characterised by apathy, lack of intiative, loss of interest (especially in things of an impersonal nature), submissiveness, apparent inability to make plans for the future, lack of individuality and sometimes a characteristic posture and gait. This occurs to the patients with chronic schizophrenia, depression, or who are elderly or organically confused.

The causes of institutional neurosis are :

(i)   loss of contact with the outside world

(ii)   enforced idleness and loss of responsibility

(iii) bossiness of medical and nursing staff

(iv)   loss of personal friends and possessions, and personal events

(v)   drugs

(vi)   ward atmosphere

(vii)   loss of prospects outside the institution

2.   Theory of social therapy

The ability of a person to live and work in an environment is a function of that part of the psychological apparatus known as the ego. It is pointed out that the need to understand psychotic and psychoneurotic illnesses and the process of psychotherapy led the psychoanalysts to study extensively the suppressed, the chaotic, the instinctual parts of the mind (the id) and the regulatory part (the superego). Social therapies are concerned with the part of mind that deals with external factors – work, other people, things – the ego. The ego has a series of ways of dealing with challenges which are called as 'sets'. The mentally retarded can have simple sets, while the intelligent and sophisticated individual can have complex sets.

3.   Social therapies in psychiatric setting

Social therapies has the basic underlying belief that the way people live in an institution that determines the extent and quality of their rehabilitation. The common themes of social therapies are:

(i)   Activity

(ii)   Freedom

(iii)   Responsibility

(i) Activity

For an unoccupied regress patient, almost any activity is good; but purposeful, socially valued, rehabilitative activity is best.

(ii) Freedom

Every bureaucratic hospital will tend to limit patient's freedom 'for fear of what may happen' and the more this extends, the more people are crippled. But freedom gives him to gain the sense of confidence and supportiveness. He perceives the psychiatric ward as non-threatening and non-punitive. It enhances free communication from him.

(iii) Responsibility

Mental hospitals tend to take away an individual's responsibility and make him passive, hostile and dependent. But giving responsibility to him helps to exercise his own assets, make his own mistakes, surmount his crisis and grow a little.

4. Living-Learning

This is another most useful concept in social therapy. This is the idea that people learn best from the things that they experience and that the incidents of everyday life should be commonly used to allow people to learn a little more about themselves and their emotions, about other people and their reactions, about what is possible and what is unacceptable in society.

Criteria to select the activity should be based on the opportunity for personal growth to greater activity, responsibility or independence. Each activity may take the patient out into the open air, give physical exercise and keep him away from the ward for a time. For example, the patient's garden often gives challenges, involves long-term planning, offers real personal achievement and the chance of earning by selling produce. It often forms a preparation for rehabilitation. —

5. Workshops

Industrial workshop activity is another method of giving social therapy. Instead of seeing groups of patients wandering aimlessly about in an airing court, or sitting mute on rows of benches, they can be engaged with love of activity and production. They are better than sitting idle and hallucinating on the ward.

The establishment of a new workshop in a locked hospital was often the first breach in a wall of indifference and was a mighty move towards liberation. It gave the patients a chance to earn money, to improve their physical circumstances and to exercise choice over areas of their lives. The patient in the workshop is engaged in a realistic task, similar to what he might do outside. He has a 'job' – which enhances his self-esteem as a member of a work-oriented society. He receives pay which he can spend on what he wants.

Social and recreational therapies hold an important and valued part in all hospitals where patients spend a long time, but especially in rehabilitation hospitals for physical medicine, and in psychiatric hospitals. They may involve in group activities – play, reading, team games, producing a paper – in which they can try out new social roles in a protected situation. For patients who are trapped in a chronic sick role, social therapy workshop may offer the only way out. The patients cannot face the abrupt transition to the full, active life of outside society. But some of this may be due to having lost some of the skills of their pre-institutional life; they can reacquire some of it like working up to a standard, coming to work on time, finishing work to a deadline, as well as the opportunity given by money to experiment with other social situations – making choices, shopping, budgeting and so on.

6. Social therapy in wards

The most important – and yet the most difficult – milieu for social therapy is the ward, the place in which the patients live. The process of social therapy in an acute ward can make their stay more understandable and less mystifying, and hasten and improve the process of return to outside life. In a long-stay ward, the aim of social therapy might be to raise the quality of the individual lives, to provide more challenges and stimuli and to re-establish connections with the family outside. In general, the social therapy can introduce the principle of 'activity', 'freedom' and 'responsibility', and then help to work towards rehabilitation and an independent life.

Communication gaps among staff, and between staff and patients is brought down through the most valuable exercise of getting the groups together to discuss mutual problems. It gives opportunity to understand the nature of problem, find solutions, modify working style and clear fantasies which they have inevitably created around each other. A conscious effort is required to change this. Individual tasks and roles must be looked at to give them a chance of improvement. Patient's initiatives must be rewarded, acceptable goals offered, and incentives held out to motivate those who seem resigned.

The goal of having social therapies in mental hospitals was often seen as preventive, negative, custodial. The aim was to prevent disasters, accidents, suicides and escapes. But the social therapy provides not only comfort and safety but also provides challenges, opportunities, and chances to make progress, to regain dignity and to get away from hospital. Festive gatherings arranged in the hospital give an occasion for people, junior staff and patients particularly, to practice unusual skills or to achieve personal humphs, it is good.

Questions

1   Define recreational therapy.

2. How do you classify recreational therapy?

3. List down the various recreation activities used in recreational therapy.

4. What are the aims of giving recreational therapy to psychiatric patients?

5. Define social therapy.

6. What is the aim of giving social therapy to psychiatric patients?

7. How do you relate social therapy with moral management of psychiatric patients?

8. Define therapeutic community.

9. What are the importance of giving social therapy to psychiatric patients?

10. How do you explain the theory of social therapy?

11. Identify the basic themes underlying social therapy.

12. How do you justify 'living-learning' concept in social therapy?

13. What is the role of 'workshops' in social therapy?

14. How does social therapy benefit in patients in psychiatric ward?

———

Occupational therapy

Occupational therapy is a potent and uniquely valuable approach to health care that enables people to take control of their own lives and overcome their own disabilities.

Occupational therapy has been described as "an active method of treatment with a profound psychological justification" (Clark, 1963). The essence of occupational therapy lies in the use of activities of every description as treatment medium, with a minimum aim of improving the quality of life and a maximum aim of complete rehabilitation.

In 1752, the Pennsylvania Hospital, Philadelphia, was established in the U.S.A., where the use of occupation as treatment for the mentally ill continued to develop until the Civil War in 1860. In December 1892, Adolf Meyer, psychiatrist reported that "the proper use of time in some helpful and gratifying activity appeared to be a fundamental issue in the treatment of the neuropsychiatric patient".

Definition

Occupation has been variously defined as "any activity which engages a person's resources of time and energy and is composed of skills and values" (Reed and Sanderson, 1980).

In 1973, Johnson defined occupation as "any goal-directed activity meaningful to the individual and providing feedback to him about his worth and value as an individual and about his inter-relatedness to others".

Occupational therapy is the application of goal-oriented, purposeful activity in the assessment and treatment of individuals with psychological, physical or developmental disabilities.

2. Major goal of occupational therapy

The main goal is to enable the patient to achieve a healthy balance of occupations through the development of skills that will allow him to function at a level satisfactory to himself and others. Sub-goals are

(i)   assess the patient's needs in terms of the occupational role required of him

(ii)   to identify the skills needed to support those roles

(iii)   to remove or minimize behaviours that interfere with occupational performance

(iv)   to improve role performance

(v)   to assist the patient to develop, relearn or maintain skills to a level of competence that will allow satisfactory performance of occupational roles

(vi)   to help the patient to perform outside the service setting at a level which will enable him to meet his needs in a way which is acceptable to himself and to society.

The focus of intervention is always the patient rather than the problem or the method of treatment.

3. Activity therapy

Activity therapy was developed for use in the area of psychosocial dysfunction or deficit, that is with people suffering from mental disorder or developmental delay.

This involves 'learning through doing', using activities that emphasize present functioning. Treatment is seen as a planned, collaborative interaction between the therapist, the patient and the environment by which new skills can be learned. It is important that the relationship between the patient and therapist is based on trust and mutual respect.

4. Process of intervention

It consists of seven stages. They are:

(i)   Initial evaluation of what patient can do and cannot do in a variety of situations over a period of time.

(ii) Development of immediate and long-term goals by patient and therapist together. Goals should be concrete and measurable so that it is easy to see when they have been reached.

(iii) Develop therapy plan with planned intervention

(iv) Implement the plan. Monitor the progress and the plan is followed until the first evaluation, if satisfactory, or altered if not.

(v)   Call for review meetings with patient and all the staff involved in treatment.

(vi) When immediate goals have been achieved set further goals and alter the treatment programme.

(vii) Highlight the monitoring when the patient is ready to discontinue treatment.

5. Areas of therapy

The most basic skills to be learned are simple task performance and group participation. Other skill areas include self-care, domestic work, recreation, productive work and intimacy.

6. Points to be kept in mind

(i) Select an activity that interests, or has the potential to interest, him.

(ii) Start at the point the patient is at and progress slowly or let him make the pace.

(iii) Provide ample reinforcement for even small achievements.

7. Approach

It uses a wide range of activities including work-oriented, recreational and creative-expressive activities. Group or individual therapy is used, depending on the needs of the patient and the therapeutic relationship is seen as a significant factor in the learning process.

8. Advantages

(i) It helps to build a more healthy and integrated ego

(ii) It helps to express and deal with needs and feelings

(iii) Assists in the gratification of frustrated basic needs

(iv)   Strengthens ego defences

(v)   Reverses psychopathology

(vi)   Facilitates personality integration

(vii) Offers opportunities to explore and re-evaluate self-concepts and object concepts

(viii) Develops a more realistic view of the self in relation to action and others.

9. Types of service

(i)   Independent living skills : self-care or self-maintenance

(ii)   Task-oriented treatment using creative-expressive modalities, crafts, education, leisure time, play, socialisation and other role-related activities

(iii) Provocational and work adjustment programmes employment and academic preparation, home making, child care or parenting

(iv)   Sensory motor, including neuromuscular and sensory-integrative assessment and treatment

(v)   Design, fabrication and application of orthotic devices

(vi)   Adaptation to physical environment and guidance in use of adaptive equipment

(vii) Therapeutic exercise to enhance functional performance

(viii) Discharge planning and community re-entry

(ix)   Patient or family education and counselling.

185

10. Settings

Occupational therapy is provided to children, adolescents, adults and the elderly of all functional groups and diagnostic categories, in institutional, community-based, partial hospitalisation, residential treatment and forensic programmes. These programmes are offered in psychiatric hospitals, nursing homes, psychosocial and physical rehabilitation centres, sheltered workshops or clinics, special schools for physically and mentally handicapped, integrated schools, community group homes, community mental health centres, day-care centres, industrial health unit, halfway homes and in de-addiction centres.

11. Occupational therapy to promote physical fitness

The activities described below have all been successfully incorporated into occupational therapy programmes for the mentally ill or mentally handicapped. They are:

(i)   Relaxation training : to 'turn off tensions'. It includes physiological techniques, meditative techniques and hypnotic techniques.

(ii) Dance : to become efficient and well co-ordinated and to function more ably in his environment.

(iii) Swimming : to enable the physically handicapped to participate as freely as the able-bodied.

(iv) Yoga : to increase concentration, stimulate interest and improve body awareness.

(v)   Keep fit : to provide accessible form of exercise with balls, hoops and ribbons.

(vi) Walking, jogging and running : to encourage people to explore their neighbourhoods and an opportunity to enjoy nature.

The broad aim of occupational therapy through physical mode is :

(a) **Physical aims**

- to improve co-ordination and spatial awareness

- to improve general physical condition and increase cardiovascular fitness

- to develop strength and suppleness and to improve posture and gait.

(b) **Personal aims**

- to improve mood and reduce anxiety

- to provide an outlet for aggressive impulses

- to improve confidence and enhance self-image

- to encourage independent personal care es pecially in dressing and grooming

- to provide opportunities for patients to face challenges and achieve success

12. Occupational therapy to enhance sensory-integration

Sensory-integrative therapy provides direct systematic and controlled therapy to remediate the underlying neural dysfunction. Enhancement of sensory-integrative function should promote more effective and adaptive occupational performance.

(i) Aims

To normalise sensory integration and therefore normalise motor and perceptual responses.

(ii) Technique

Non-competitive pleasurable activities are used to reduce anxiety, which interferes with sensory integration in the reticular and limbic systems by producing over-arousal.

(iii) Treatment activities

Kicking and throwing balls

Rolling

Crawling

Scooter board

Hopping

Skipping

Jumping

These activities improve body image, and spatial and form perception.

13. Occupational therapy for developing cognitive skills

It is given to increase the capacity of the patient to perform tasks competently and to fulfill his normal life roles.

(i) Aims

- to restore the lost skills; for example, practicing cookery after a head injury

- to use remaining skills to compensate for the loss; for example, learning to make lists to compensate for loss of memory

- to make adjustments in life-style so that the lost skills are not needed; for example, moving into a hostel where meals will be provided

Cognitive skills are taught as an integral part of achieving competence in occupational performance.

(ii) Treatment activities

- Crafts, which are useful for developing concentration, creative thinking and planning

- Quizzes and table games, for developing concentration memory, and problem-solving skills

- Art and poetry, for developing creative thinking and imagination

- Play-reading or discussion, to develop language skills, concentration and memory

- Creative writing, to develop creative thinking, language skills and concept formation

- Reality orientation, to develop memory, attention, concentration and orientation

14. Classification of occupational therapy

Occupational therapy may be diversional (e.g., organised games which stimulate spontaneity and freedom of movement and the competitiveness and excitement tends to take away the patient's anxious preoccupation with the diseased part) or remedial (physiotherapy for particular muscle groups, e.g., basket making, carpentry, embroidery, gardening) physiotherapy (which includes heat massage, electrotherapy, remedial exercises either assisted by the therapist or free or resisted by weights, pulleys, etc.) is used with the main emphasis on rehabilitation.

15. Occupational therapy in an in-patient unit

Occupational therapy programme usually consists of a wide range of both individual and group experiences designed to meet the patient's social, emotional, and occupational needs based on the abilities of the patients, (activities like craft work, sewing, leather work, ceramics and wood work and weaving).

Beyond this, these programmes offer assertiveness training, daily living skills groups and current event groups. Art range activities, including music, art, clay work, poetry and drama are given to patients in group as an explorative measure, providing ways of bringing people together and exploring the self. Painting is used as a vehicle for self-expression. For chronic long-stay patients, the therapeutic interventions are training for physical wellbeing, daily living skills, social activities, social skills training, creative activities, craft activities and industrial work.

Questions

1. Define occupational therapy.

2. List the major therapeutic goals of giving occupational therapy to psychiatric patients.

3. Define activity therapy.

4. What are the process of intervention involved in an activity therapy?

5. Identify the areas of activity therapy.

6. What do you keep in mind while selecting an activity to a psychiatric patient?

7. What are the advantages of activity therapy?

8. Discuss the types of services provided through activity therapy.

9. Identify the activities incorporated in occupational therapy to promote physical fitness in patients.

10. Mention the broad aims of giving occupational therapy to psychiatric patients.

11. How do you enhance sensory integration through occupational therapy to psychiatric patients?

12. How does cognitive skills develop through occupational therapy?

13. How do you classify occupational therapy?

14. How does occupational therapy is being implemented in the in-patient unit of mental hospitals?

_____

191

Legal aspects of psychiatric nursing

In no other type of nursing are the legal and ethical considerations of practice so crucial as in psychiatric nursing. To deal with these demands, psychiatric nurses must be aware of both the laws in the state in which they practice and the common practice of nurses in the area. Law addresses the outcome of behaviour and has developed a system of rules and regulations to facilitate orderly social functioning. The practice of psychiatric nursing is influenced by the law, particularly in its concern for the rights of patients and the quality of care they are receiving.

In the history of law, nurses have been protected from direct suits by patients because of the perception that they are either dependent on the physician or employees of an institution for orders. Attorneys sue directly the physician or the hospital rather than the nurse. Now, with the advent of consumerism, the recognition of professional nursing as an independent discipline and the awareness that all nurses register with their state nursing council to practice nursing, there is an increase demand to get well-versed with legal aspects of psychiatric nursing.

Nurses are bounded with Nurse Practice Act. It defines nursing only as "the administration of medications and treatment as is prescribed by a licensed physician".

It is a service that could be considered dependent for the nurse; that is, it is dependent on the acts (orders) of someone else. The rest of the mandated activities are acts that the nurse can, should and must do on her own initiative because patients need and should reasonably expect these nursing actions. Nurses are responsible and accountable for these nursing acts and are responsible for performing them in a manner that is safe for the patient.

Nursing malpractice

It is important to define nursing malpractice. Malpractice is a professional negligence. Malpractice is a civil action that can be brought against a nurse if she has breached a standard of care that a reasonably prudent nurse would meet.

Malpractice is a kind of tort action that is brought by a consumer plaintiff against a defendant professional from whom the consumer plaintiff feels that he has received injury during the course of the professional-consumer relationship.

In order for a plaintiff consumer to receive money damages by successfully suing a professional nurse for malpractice, the consumer plaintiff must prove the following five elements of nursing negligence :

(i)   the nurse professional had a duty to use due care towards the plaintiff.

(ii)   the nurse professional's performance fell below the standard of care and was therefore a breach of that duty.

(iii) as a result of the failure to meet the standard of care, the plaintiff consumer was injured and the nurse's action was the proximate cause of the injury.

(iv)   the act that the nurse engaged in could foreseeably have caused an injury.

(v)   the plaintiff consumer must prove his injuries.

In a malpractice action against the nurse, the proof of the standard of care becomes an essential and important ingredient. As nurses are being held increasingly responsible and monetarily liable for nursing practice and malpractice, nursing must and will take control of nursing practice issues such as staffing, educational qualifications and competencies and role definition on the health care team.

Quality patient care provided by nursing greatly decreases malpractice litigation and successful recovery against both professional and corporate defendants. And, of course, quality patient care can only be legally proved by clear, concise, accurate, complete and outcome-oriented documentation. The medical record is the best source of legal protection in a malpractice suit.

Informed consent

All patients have a right to informed consent prior to health care interventions. The performance of health care treatments or procedures without the informed consent of the patient can result in legal action against the physician and the health care agency.

Consent is an absolute defense to battery, and informed consent is required in health care situations. Battery is a touching of the person of another, of his clothes, or anything else attached to his person without consent. Informed consent can be defined as that knowing consent that is given in an interaction or series of interactions between the treating physician and the patient that allows the patient to fully consider information about the treatment that is being proposed (e.g., the way it will be administered, its prognosis, its side effects, its risks, the possible consequences of refusing the treatment, and other treatment alternatives).

A major problem with consent arises with psychiatric patients because the validity of their competence to agree to a procedure is usually questioned. Many mental patients are capable of giving informed consent. They are aware of their surroundings, they understand what is being said, they are making their decisions based on what they think is best for them, and they are doing it without coercion. But some psychiatric patients are with gross impairments and they do not understand what is being said and are therefore unable to give valid consent. Because of this unreliability, major nursing considerations in the psychiatric nursing practice area of informed consent are the constant monitoring and observing of patients for the following :

(i) a state of legal capacity or competence when they are asked to give informed consent.

(ii) continuing understanding of the information that they have been given.

(iii) power and opportunities to revoke consent at any time during a particular course of treatment

Substituted consent

When it is determined that a patient is unable to give informed consent, providers of health services should obtain substituted consent for the necessary treatment or procedure.

Substitute consent is that authorisation given by another person on behalf of one who is in need of a procedure or treatment. Substituted consent can come from a court-appointed guardian or in some instances, from the patient's next of kin. If the kin is not available, the health care agency may initiate a court proceeding to appoint a guardian so that the procedure or treatment can be carried out.

It is important for nurses, along with other health care providers, to know the statutory requirements for obtaining substituted consent. It is also necessary for the nurse functioning in the role of patient advocate to know whether a patient has been adjudicated incompetent and whether consent from a next of kin or a guardian is a legally acceptable substitution for the consent of the patient. Assuring legally adequate informed consent prior to treatment should be an important part of the psychiatric nursing care plan.

Confidentiality

In nursing practice, it is well acknowledged that the information gathered about the patient through interpersonal relationships and from indirect sources are both confidential. It is a professional and an ethical duty to use the knowledge that is gained about patients for the enhancement of their care rather than for other purposes, such as gossip, personal gain, or mere curiosity. The confidentiality of verbal, as well as written material must be maintained.

Stigma attached to mental illness is still prevailing. Any breach of confidentiality of data/information about patients, their diagnoses, their symptoms, their behaviours, and the outcomes of treatment can certainly affect the course of the rest of their lives in terms of employment, promotions, marriage, attainment of insurance benefits and so forth. Psychiatric nurses have to take care for keeping the information regarding patients confidential.

Responsible record keeping

Records are legal documents that can be used in court; therefore, all nursing notes and progress record should reflect descriptive, non-judgmental and objective statements. Examples of significant data include here-and-now observations of the patient through the use of the nurse's senses, accurate reporting of what is said and what is done for the patient, and a description of the outcomes of the care provided.

Verbal communications and data sharing are important, especially on treatment terms and units that use multidisciplinary approaches to patient care. The verbal sharing should be straightforward, forthright, descriptive and unopinionated, and shared only with those individuals who are involved in the care and treatment of the patient.

Basic rights of psychiatric patients and nurse's responsibility.

It is the responsibility of the nurses to ensure that their actions promote the welfare of patients. Psychiatric patients are often the least capable of protecting their own rights. Psychiatric problems may cause patients to lack social skills or may cause an inability to make a point clearly understood because of difficulties in concentration. As a result, the rights of psychiatric patients have been ignored and abused for centuries.

When a psychiatric patient enters a hospital, he loses his freedom to come and go, to schedule his day, to choose his activities, and to control his activities of daily living. If he is also adjudicated incompetent, he loses his freedom to manage his financial and legal affairs and make many important decisions. Because of the loss of these important freedoms, the authorities of health care agencies closely guard and value those rights that the psychiatric patient retains. Some of the rights of the psychiatric patients are:

(i)   the right to wear their own clothes.

(ii)   the right to keep and use their own personal possessions, including toilet articles.

(iii)   the right to keep and be allowed to spend a reasonable sum of their money for canteen expenses and small purchases.

(iv)   the right to have access to individual storage space for their private use.

(v)   the right to see visitors every day.

(vi)   the right to have reasonable access to telephones, both to make and to receive calls.

(vii)   the right to have ready access to letter-writing materials.

(viii)   the right to mail and receive unopened correspondence.

(ix)   the right to refuse electroconvulsive therapy.

(x)   the right to manage and dispose of property.

(xi)   the right to execute wills.

(xii)   the right to hold civil service status.

(xiii)   the right to treatment in the least restrictive setting.

Nursing has long espoused a philosophy that one of its important roles in the health care system is to act as an advocate for the patient. The advocacy role is nowhere more important than in the psychiatric care system as an assessor of, nd spokesman for, the protection of patient's rights.

Discussing rights within treatment teams, including these rights in the nursing care plan, and ensuring that methodologies for rights protection are nursing activities that fulfill the role as patient's advocate. One important resource that nursing should request is ongoing legal advice and consultation in the area of patient's rights. These are mostly prescribed and governed by health care agency in India.

However, to protect patient's rights, the nurses should be made aware of patient's rights, ensure that ward procedure and policy does not violate patient's rights, review periodically the rights, issues of violations, and mechanisms that provide rights accountability and specifically review the changes in voluntary, involuntary status, civil or criminal commitment proceedings and treatment consequences.

Voluntary patients may seek treatment and the non-dangerous involuntary patients may not be confined without treatment. But those treatments need to be and occur in methods and settings that are least restrictive to the patient's liberty. Involuntary patients who are non-dangerous have limited rights to refuse medication and have greater rights to refuse more invasive procedures such as ECT. Competence to consent and procedures for substituted consent are always at issue with involuntarily committed patients. These legal issues have to be borne in mind while working with psychiatric patients.

Legal responsibilities of a mentally ill person

Responsibility in the legal sense means the liability of a person for his acts or omissions and if such be contrary to law, the liability to be punished for them.

(i) Criminal responsibility

Section 84 of the Indian Penal Code of 1860 provides that "nothing is an offence which is done by a person who, at the time of doing it by reason of unsoundness of mind, was incapable of knowing the nature of the act or that what he was doing was either wrong or contrary to law". The phase of insanity is generally brought forward during the trial stage. The accused is found not guilty, if insanity is established.

An Amendment (1957) that includes irresistible impulses (covered under irresistible insanity) which are beyond the control of the lunatic is incorporated under section 84 of Indian Penal Code.

Irresistible impulse test is used along with M'Naghten rule. It is never used in isolation. According to this test, a person may know the difference between right and wrong but finds himself impulsively driven to commit the criminal act. It is usually necessary to snow a lack of premeditation and that the urge was so strong that it would have been followed regardless of the circumstances. This test is frequent defense for sudden, violent behaviour displayed under stress.

This concept is based on M' Naghten Rule. This law originated with the 1832 London trial of Daniel M' Naghten when he was tried for the murder of Edward Drummond, private secretary of Sir Robert Peele. M'

Naghten had suffered from delusions of persecution and had complained to public authorities many times. Receiving no help, however, he decided to resolve the situation himself. He began watching the house of Sir Robert Peele and one evening, under the belief he was shooting Peele, shot Edward Drummond as he emerged from the house. His attorney Mr. Cockburn defended M' Naghten. Justice Tindall was the judge. M' Naghten was declared of unsound mind and committed to an institution for the criminally insane. In deciding the case, the judge identified two rules to determine the criminal responsibility of a person who pleads insanity.

The first rule states that the individual at the time of the crime did not "know the nature and quality of act".

The second states that if he did not know what he was doing, he did not know that it "was wrong". These two rules are called the "nature and quality" rule and "right from wrong" test. This case was the first major test of criminal responsibility and it is still used in criminal courts.

(ii)   Durham Rule (1954)

"An accused person is not criminally responsible if his unlawful act is the product of mental disease or mental defect". In this, the causal connection between the mental abnormality and the alleged crime should be established. This broad standard of causality referred to as the "but-for-cause" standard would free almost all defendants who could show any degree of mental disease or defect. It has not gained wide acceptance.

This rule is based on 'Durham test' or "Product rule". The Durham test is based on a 1954 decision in the District of Columbia. The rule states that the accused is not criminally responsible if his act was the "product of mental disease". Thus it is sometimes called the "Product Rule".

(iii) American Law Institute's (ALI) test

"A person is not responsible for criminal conduct if at the time of such conduct as a result of mental disease or defect he lacks adequate capacity either to appreciate the criminality of his conduct or to conform his conduct to the requirements of the law".

This ALI test is similar to the combination of the M' Naguten Rule and Irresistible Impulse Test. It excludes "an abnormality manifested only by repeated criminal or otherwise antisocial conduct", which excludes the psychopath who has repeated criminal conduct. This popular test is now used by all courts.

Similarly the persons with Somnambulism, and impulse because of insanity, delirium or involuntary drunkenness are also not criminally responsible.

Civil responsibility

A person has no responsibility in the following conditions, if he is proved to be a lunatic.

(i) Management of property and affairs of insane

On the application of any relative of an alleged lunatic, the court may direct an inquiry to ascertain whether the person is of unsound mind and incapable of managing his property and affairs. The medical evidence is given in the form of a certificate, which should state "the insanity is of such a degree as to render him incapable of managing his property and affairs". In case of doubt, it is safer to give an opinion in favour of sanity. In case of insanity, the court appoints a manager to look after his property, granting him necessary powers (e.g. sale or disposal of the lunatic's property for payment of his debts and expenses), until the insanity has ceased. Under the Transfer of Property Act (1982), only persons competent to contract are authorised to transfer property.

(iii) Marriage

Under the Hindu Marriage Act (1955) a marriage between two parties, either of whom was of unsound mind at the time of the marriage is considered void. Divorce can be obtained on the ground of incurable unsoundness of mind for a specific continuous period. If lunacy starts after marriage and continues for 2 years even with treatment, the other party can apply for legal separation and if the illness continues for more than three years, then the other party can apply for divorce but the other party has to pay for the maintenance of the lunatic. This is for all cases when the other party is male and in certain cases, when the other party is female.

(iii) Testamentary capacity (testament=will)

Indian Succession Act 1925 refers as testamentary capacity to the mental ability of a person to make a valid will.

The requirements for a valid will are as follows

(a)   A written and properly signed   and   witnessed

instrument must exist. The testator must be major, and free of any force, undue influence or dishonest representation of facts applied by others at the time of the signing of the will. Doctors or nurses are sometimes called upon to witness the execution of the will of an ailing person. The testator is said to be of sound mind if he is capable of disposing of his property with understanding and reason. The tests used for this purpose by a doctor include tests for orientation, memory, concentration, and for the nature, extent and value of his properties and manner of its distribution. He should be asked in the absence of all attendants, whether any pressure or influence has been brought on him by any one.

(b)   Persons affected by an insane delusion can make a valid will if the delusion is not related in any way to the disposal of the property, or the persons affected by the will. Persons can make valid wills during lucid interval. Prejudices, dislikes and antipathies, however ill founded or strongly entertained, cannot be classed as insane delusion. Partial drunkenness or the extremes of the ages do not invalid a contract, if the reasoning powers are intact.

(iv) Election or right of vote

No person of unsound mind can contest election or exercise the franchise of voting. A person can be debarred from contesting election or by exercising a vote by the court.

The legal impact on the practice of psychiatric nursing is both immense and subtle. The psychiatric nurse who evaluates her practice in an attempt to improve the nursing profession and the health of her patients does so not from legal demands but from professional standards. Nevertheless, nursing practice must meet certain legal standards and must adjust its course as new legal standards evolve. It is the capable and challenged nurse who includes legal knowledge in patient care and it is to her that many patients will turn for information, advocacy, and protective justice.

Questions

1. Explain the legal aspects of psychiatric nursing.

2. What is the role of psychiatric nurse in maintaining the basic rights of psychiatric patients?

3. Discuss the criminal responsibility in psychiatric nursing.

4. Write short notes on :

    i) M'Naghten rule

    ii) Testamentary capacity

    iii) Civil rights of mentally ill

    iv) Nursing mal practice.

Rehabilitation

Rehabilitation services are designed to prevent chronic disability. It provides the opportunity to acquire and maintain the life skills that are necessary to cope effectively. Rehabilitation involves helping the handicapped people to attain their best level of social functioning, which for some people means a fully independent life, and for others (those with severe impairments) life-long support. Good rehabilitation requires skilled assessment of each patient's potential, a wide range of treatment methods and continuity of care.

The public health model of prevention includes three levels of preventive health care activity : primary, secondary, and tertiary. **Primary prevention** focuses on decreasing the number of new cases (incidence) of a health problem by intervening before an illness occurs. **Secondary prevention** focuses on prompt intervention when illness occurs to limit the length and severity of an episode. **Tertiary prevention** is the limitation of disability related to an episode of an illness.

Any episode of illness may involve lasting change in the individual's level of functioning. A person who has been more seriously ill is more likely to have serious problems living productively in the community. Hospitalisation is especially disruptive to the person's life, and it is difficult to adjust after discharge. Nurses working in the hospital setup must be aware of the total range of the present and potential patient care needs.

Definition

Rehabilitation is the process of enabling the individual to return to his highest possible level of functioning. The goal is usually to exceed the pre-illness functional level. This may be achieved by assisting the patients to regain their strengths, relearning the old skills, or learning new skills depending on the effects of the health care problem and the person's response to it.

Maxwell Jones defined rehabilation as "the attempt to provide the best possible community role which will enable the patient to achieve the maximum range of activity, compatible with his personality, interests and of which he is capable."

The major task in rehabilitation is the reconstruction of the patient's ego strengths so that he can be made mentally fit and ready for work and also able to cope with the emotional and interpersonal factors involved in starting and continuing on the job. Rehabilitation is also a philosophy – an attitude – a state of mind – a mode of approach to illness.

Rehabilitation is a process of minimizing psychiatric impairments, social disadvantages and adverse personal reactions, so that the disabled person is helped to use his or her talents and to acquire confidence and self-esteem through experiencing success in social roles. It should be distinguished from resettlement, which is a simpler concept meaning just what it says – replacing a person into a particular setting, usually from sheltered day facilities, to work.

Certain principles have been identified as basic to most psychiatric rehabilitation settings. They are as follows:

i)   The primary focus is on the improvement of the capabilities and the competence of the person with psychiatric problems, even the most disabled. The alleviation of symptoms is secondary.

ii) Insight is not a primary goal; rather, this focuses on the ability to function.

iii) Utilises a variety of therapeutic constructs.

iv) Improvement of vocational outcomes is a central focus.

v)   Emphasis on positive expectations and hope is essential to the process.

vi) A deliberate increase in dependency, as in sheltered settings, may be a first step in the process.

vii) Active participation and involvement of patients in rehabilitation.

viii) Patient skill development and environmental resource development and, fundamental interventions in the rehabilitation process.

Thus, the comprehensive network of services recognises and emphasises continuity of care, with an indefinite time frame.

Psychiatric rehabilitation approaches have also been termed psychosocial treatments. There are a few trends seen in psychosocial treatment, namely,

i)   **Psychoeducation** includes diagnosing the problem, telling the person what to expect from the illness and discussing treatment alternatives.

An important function of psychoeducational work is to identify hitherto unspoken fears and to correct myths and prejudices by providing basic information in a context of respect and hope.

ii) **Working with families** includes utilising the resources of family towards the welfare of patient. Families are involved in treatment and rehabilitation programme as partners in providing care.

iii) **Group therapy** : For many severely mentally disabled people, group treatment is more effective than individual therapy. Positive aspects of group therapy include an opportunity for ongoing contact with others, validation of their perceptions, sharing their views about problem and problem solving abilities and intensity of participation.

iv) **Social skills** : It involves teaching specific living skills that the patient is expected to need to survive in a community setting. It focuses on the abilities required for normal social interaction like making conversation, expressing feelings, employment skills, management of money and reduction of socially embarrassing behaviour such as intrusiveness and poor hygiene.

Acceptance of the cured patient by the family and the community

The rehabilitation process of psychiatric patients must be evaluated in relation to the patient's milieu, the family's tolerance to his psychological defects, the sense of responsibility and orientation of the therapeutic team in various forms of assistance, and the solidarity and continuity of study in the care of illness.

Rehabilitation is viewed as a series of progressive stages of which we are concerned with two – one in which the patient is able to succeed in remaining in the community and a second in which he is able not only to stay in the community but to attain as well a level of occupational and social functioning comparable to that of most other adult members of the community.

Difficulties in rehabilation

The period of readjustment to community life can be an extremely difficult and traumatic one for the person who has been hospitalised for mental illness. Patients released from a mental hospital frequently encounter two typical problems:

i) to find adequate housing in a wholesome environment, and

ii) to find work.

Some persons in the complex urban society are unable to maintain themselves in the larger community and unable to participate occupationally and socially in the life of that community.

There is little doubt that residence in the community and participation in its activities are accorded high values by a large sector of our society as the only appropriate life way for the adult individual; and this is certainly true of the values held by members of mental health professions as well as by other groups concerned with community welfare. The community tenure of former patients has been used as an indicator of the efficacy of new therapies as a dependent variable in the study of correlates of mental illness, and as the critical factor in planning for additional personnel and bed space in hospitals. Despite diversity of definitions of rehabilitation there is virtual agreement among psychiatric practitioners that, at the very minimum, the rehabilitated patient must be able to live in a non-medical setting.

There are two types of functions in the family group – 'instrumental' and 'expressive' functions. An instrumental function is one primarily concerned with the relations of the group to the situation external to it, including adaptation to the conditions of that situation and establishment of satisfactory goal relations for the system vis-a-vis the situations. Expressive function on the other hand is concerned – primarily with the harmony or solidarity of the group, the relations internally of the members to each other and their emotional states of tension or lack of it in their roles in the group.

How far the discharged mental patient is able to perform these instrumental and expressive roles within and outside the family, largely depends upon the attitudes shown by his family members and the community.

Adequate occupational and social performance is at least one of the ways in which healthy and sick individuals are differentiated. There is an emphasis on instrumental role performance because it is culturally valued and thought to have social utility even within the hospital setting.

The post-hospital fate of the mental patient can be described along with variety of dimensions. Perhaps the most critical dimension is success or failure in remaining in the community, which we consider the first stage in rehabilitation.

Process of rehabilitation for a cured patient

It involves three stages or phases:

(i)   Psychiatric rehabilitation

(ii) Social rehabilitation

(iii) Vocational rehabilitation

For the psychiatric patient, rehabilitation involves developing an adjustment to himself (insight), to his family and friends and to the community in which he plans to reside.

Psychiatric rehabilitation

It places the patient in a programme of direct treatment which may take one or more different forms like chemotherapy, social therapy, etc.

Social rehabilitation

It focuses on developing desirable social relationships (both within and outside the hospital). The patient has to be adequately prepared for the major task he has to face, a breaking through different layers of social barriers on his return to life in the community.

The emphasis is on his restoration of ability to take roles adequately expected of him in the family, community and society at large. This may involve relearning of healthy role taking and unlearning of deviant roles the ex-patient is performing.

Thus, social rehabilitation is an important aspect of social psychiatry which is defined – "social psychiatry refers to the preventive and curative measures which are directed towards the fitting of the individual for a satisfactory and useful life in terms of his own social-environment". In order to achieve this goal, opportunity for making contacts with society which are favourable to the maintenance or re-establishment of social adequacy are of prime importance for the mentally ill, and for those in danger of becoming so.

Vocational rehabilitation

It provides the patient with such specialised services as counselling and vocational guidance, vocational training, development of adequate work tolerance and work-social skills, job-finding, specialised psychological testing, selecting job placement and adequate vocational follow-up services.

All three phases of rehabilitation must mesh smoothly and purposefully in a common cause from the very onset of treatment, through discharge and follow-up of services. The independence of the phases of rehabilitation cannot be overstressed, nor can any one of them be considered less important than the others.

Generally speaking, those who are inadequate, insecure, immature, neurotic and psychopathic will have more difficulty in making the best use of their residual resources; these are the poorer rehabilitation risks. The mature, well-adjusted person is the better rehabilitation risk.

The feelings of insecurity, inadequacy and such others are the results of the inter-personal, intra-familial environment of the patient right from the childhood. It may be related to premorbid period post-recovery period, the period of illness either singly or in combination. The role

213

of attitudes of relatives is of vital importance in making the individual's healthy growth.

To be successful, the rehabilitation of the mentally ill patient must be thought of as a continuum which must begin, at least from the stand point of evaluation and planning, from the moment the patient enters the hospital, clinic or private office. He must pass through successive levels of development until he is able to be reintegrated into society and employment. He must be thought of as a "totality" (psychiatrically, vocationally and socially) as early as possible after the beginning of treatment. This implies the importance of team work composed of psychiatrists, psychologists, social workers, nurses and relatives.

Attitudes of relatives affect the patient after discharge in subtle ways and are deciding factors in keeping the patient out of or in the hospital. Each patient has different levels of adjustment to his environment. There are mainly three levels of adjustment.

In the first level, the patient is well adjusted socially, emotionally and occupationally as a gainful member of the society. But negative attitudes of relatives may precipitate the attack. Therefore, modification of attitudes may avoid relapse, help in preventing those who are in danger of becoming so and last but not least in preserving and promoting the mental health of the society.

In the second level, the patient is fairly well adjusted but has some minor difficulties. If these are not attended to in time, the problems will be accentuated, causing relapse. Hence timely help with acceptance and positive, sympathetic attitude will arrest further deterioration.

In the third level, the patient is in the community but is a burden to the family and community at large. The patient also will be suffering for want of proper treatment and positive attitude and acceptance. If treated, such patients will not become chronic.

Hence the acceptance of cured psychiatric patients by family and community becomes very essential. Several helpful approaches of nurses to families have been identified. They are:

(i)   allow the family members to express their feelings about the patient's illness and how it relates to their lives.

(ii)   provide the information that families need to participate in decision making.

(iii)   assist them to deal with the feelings of apprehension, worries about the patient.

(iv)   identify the coping method that is being used and assess its helpfulness. Families with mental illness may try to cope with the patient by denying the seriousness of the problem, by being over-controlling or by withdrawing.

(v)   help the family to learn to balance their own needs with those of the patient.

Similarly, there are several ways that nurses can intervene in the community to encourage the establishment of tertiary prevention programmes for psychiatric patients. It will enable the community to express its acceptance towards the cured mental patients.

Social networks in the community could extend its services through,

(i)   emotional support

(ii)   task-oriented assistance

(iii)   communication of expectations, evaluations

(iv)   access to social contact

Re-employment

Many action-oriented programmes resulting from systematic exploration of the rehabilitation potentials are being initiated and implemented for the welfare of the blind, deaf-mute, and orthopaedically handicapped. For example, there are 13 vocational rehabilitation centres organised by the Ministry of Labour, Employment and Training, Government of India, functioning in different state capitals which deal with the problems of the physically handicapped. Even the special employment exchanges are concerned with the welfare of the physically handicapped. But, in the case of mentally disabled who are either mentally ill or mentally retarded, only sporadic attempts are made to fully utilise the inherent potentials. Unfortunately, there is neither special employment exchange nor any vocational rehabilitation centre for the welfare of the mentally disabled persons.

In the absence of necessary vocational training facilities leading to vocational rehabilitation either in the mental hospital setting or community settings, the mentally disabled persons become more and more dependent on the families which in turn are increasingly frustrated with these individuals, and ultimately such unhealthy chain reactions resulting in patients being thrown out of the families. Thus wandering becomes their main activity, begging becomes their vocation and public's mockery becomes reward from the society. Specially when the mentally ill happens to be the head of the family or the only bread winner of the family, lack of vocational rehabilitation programmes may lead to·untold miseries. The plight of the children and helpless wife are pathetic. The family gets totally disorganised -- young children forced to give up their schooling in order to earn their livelihood through hard child labour; wife, if not supported by either the relatives or social security measures, becomes the personification of sadness and hopelessness. Such family situations, more often than not, become the target of anti-social elements too.

Mainly three categories of mentally disabled could be identified from the vocational rehabilitation point of view. They are:

(i) persons who lost their jobs because of the disease process.

(ii) individuals who were deprived of education and training opportunities owing to the early onset of illness.

(iii) patients who were left with residual psychiatric problems affecting their vocational career.

Successful vocational rehabilitation programmes for these three categories of the disabled persons largely depend on the compliance to the physical rehabilitation (drug treatment) and psychosocial rehabilitation aiming at improvement of the individual's psychological conditions and social environment.

The International Labour Organisation (ILO - 1979) formulated the principles of vocational rehabilitation of the mentally restored. Mentally restored is defined as a person who is recovering or has recovered from mental illness and he/she is ready to receive vocational assistance including vocational preparation and evaluation, and vocational training leading to employment in the open labour market or under sheltered conditions.

The principles of vocational rehabilitation are as follows:

(i)　In the rehabilitation process, not only the disability itself but also the residual abilities and social circumstances of the disabled should be taken into account as early as possible.

(ii)　In the overall field of rehabilitation, the educational element is particularly important if rehabilitation is to be regarded as a process of social learning.

(iii)　It is considered imperative that wherever possible, a mentally ill or mentally restored person should maintain contact with the network of social relationships in his home area.

(iv)　Uniform access to rehabilitation services must be provided at the local level and in such a way that the relevant involvement of the hospital, local employment offices and the general or sheltered employment markets is well coordinated.

(v)　At the national level, those health, labour, social and other services participating in the rehabilitation process should be interconnected.

(vi)　Vocational rehabilitation services for mentally restored should be integrated, wherever possible, with those for the physically disabled.

(vii)　The aims and objectives of rehabilitation programmes are generally attained only if medical treatment is integrated with a structured programme of various rehabilitation services.

(viii) It is necessary to create a legal framework to ensure job security for the disabled and facilitate vocational resettlement, independent of the economic situation.

The goal of reintegration of the mentally restored into the community could be achieved through the following four means:

(i) Open competitive job placement

Though it is difficult to place the mentally restored in the open competitive job placements, it is not impossible to provide this opportunity for the selected groups of patients with the clinical diagnosis of reactive psychosis, manic-depressive psychosis with infrequent attacks, and acute psychotic episodes. They would be able to function successfully with their duties, of course, with regular follow-up programmes.

(ii) Sheltered employment

This is provided for those disabled persons who because of the nature and severity of the disability cannot cope with ordinary employment. This is suitable for those with the problems of mental retardation, and chronic illness (Schizophrenia, repeated attacks of affective disorder inspite of regular medication, etc.).

(iii) Self-employment

Persons who cannot cope with the demands of vocational adjustment in the open competitive job situations, but who have the capacity to do some work with the help of any family member could be considered for self-employment schemes which are usually sponsored by different welfare schemes of the nationalised banks and social welfare departments. The uniqueness of this method of re-employment or vocational rehabilitation is that because of the involvement of the family members, not only the work output and income improve but also the feelings of acceptance and security are strengthened among the mentally restored persons, mentally retarded and persons with residual schizophrenia and certain categories of manic depressive psychosis.

(iv) Home-bound work programmes

Mentally disabled persons with the categories mentioned in the self-employment rehabilitation programmes can also be considered to do the work for the units set up by the small-scale industrialists and welfare organisations. Advantages of this method are, firstly, there is no need of financial investment on the part of the family members and secondly, the problems relating to the marketing of the products are absent.

Vocational rehabilitation in India is based on the setting of urban and rural and the rehabilitation potentials availability in the family and community. Because of feeling of acceptance, and patients doing some work or other related to agriculture, the rural areas offer better rehabilitation scope than the urban areas where high skills and preparation are needed for any job.

Hence, the vast potentials of rehabilitation in rural setting could be used and a variety of assignments could be given to the individuals depending on the capacity. If he is mentally retarded simple tasks like gardening, fetching the grass or grazing the cattle or other crafts would be given. If he is chronic mental patient, he could be asked to help in the household activities, keeping the cattleshed clean, taking food to the people working in the field and other work which he is capable of doing. This is the therapeutic setup that could be made available in the natural setting even for the mentally restored ·people.

In urban community, re-employment opportunities could be strengthened either by insisting large industries; both in public sector (central and state) and private sector undertakings to reserve a minimum of 20% of their light engineering assemblies for sub-contract to sheltered workshops from their present and future expanded capacities. All manufacturing/subcontracting industries established for rehabilitation of disabled people should be exempted from all taxes and the Government should ensure supply of all essential and scarce raw materials and also availability of concessional finance from banks for running those units effectively.

Incentives by way of 100% income tax exemption should be made available to all the sub-contracting industries from all earnings as a result of sub-contracting to sheltered workshops.

Voluntary agencies/organisations are to be involved in the rehabilitation programmes based in the hospital and in the community. Complete income-tax exemption should be given to all such donations to the rehabilitation measures of the disabled. To the job reservation quota of 3% for the disabled, a 1% quota must be added for the mentally disabled. Family pension could be extended to the families of mentally ill. Subsidized transport facilities and travel concessions could be provided as it is being provided for the physically disabled. Social Welfare Departments should have a separate Directorate for disabilities which should include mental disabilities also. A separate cell to be established in the Health Directorate of Central and State Governments for rehabilitation programmes for the mentally disabled.

Several chronic mentally ill patients and the mentally restored patients need long-term vocational rehabilitation programmes in the community to become self-governed re-employed people.

Follow-up

Patients, their families and every one in the treating team need to be aware that recovery has only begun when an in-patient or out-patient programme is completed. The few months immediately following completion of a treatment programme are dangerous for the mentally restored person. Relapse is not uncommon. For this reason follow-up care is essential.

The success of any mental health programme should not be measured by the number of new cases detected, but rather by the number of patients, who, duly diagnosed, continue their treatment to its end. A study of follow-up pattern reveals facts relating to community's or family's perception of mental illness. It also serves as an indirect evaluation of the impact of the initial therapeutic strategies and the multifarious problems faced by the patients and their relatives in maintaining such follow-up.

In general psychiatric clinics 20% to 57% of the patients fail to return after the first visit and 31 to 36%, attend no more than four times (Dodd, 1971). More than one-third of the mentally ill persons do not keep up the psychiatric appointment after brief evaluation and another third drop out after detailed initial evaluation, thus leaving only a third of the identified population with problem to utilise the presently limited existing psychiatric facilities (Srinivas Murthy et al 1974 and 1977).

Follow-up programme is a linking programme between intensive treatment and a complete cessation of treatment. This is designed to help the patient to gradually withdraw from the treatment process and to get himself adjusted to the family environment from where he had gone for the hospital treatment either as in-patient or out-patient. But the patients, whether in-patients or out-patients are found to be not making use of the follow-up services to the extent they are expected to. This could be due to various reasons. The initial treatment itself may not be to their expectation or to their choice or the outcome may not be a successful one.

Many studies conducted in this area revealed the following areas related to the source of problems of the families who were not able to continue the treatment.

(i)   High expectations of the family members. Eg: Fast recovery and good prognosis, etc.

(ii)   Patient refused to take oral drugs and thereby no meaning in coming for the follow-up visit to hospital to get re-prescribed with medicines.

(iii)   Excessive emotional involvement with the patient.

(iv)   Lack of understanding of patient's residual symptoms.

(v)   Problems related to marriage.

(vi)   Fear of social stigma hampered regular visit to the clinic.

(vii) Lack of understanding about illness and the importance of regular medication.

Some of the suggestions given below would help to improve treatment adherence and regular follow-up.

(i) Treating team must establish a good relationship with patients and family members and inform adequately about their illness, treatment procedure, and possible side effects of the drugs.

An orientation given in the first visit itself will enhance the follow-up.

(ii) Family members or close relatives must be involved to supervise and dispense the medication regularly. Nurses could play a major role in invoiving the family members in patient care.

(iii) Emotional, social, practical and financial advice/guidance support from family members, close relatives, friends and colleagues to the patients will enhance the treatment adherence.

(iv) For enhancing the regularity in follow-up, the health personnel, especially nurses, should followup the patients regularly. Whenever the patient is staying far away from the health care institution or in an interior village, the nurses and the health assistants should dispense the drugs. In case of any complication with drugs or any problem with disease, they should direct the patients to the nearby health care institutions.

(v) Regular education to the patient's families about the illnesses and the mportance of regular followup will increase the follow-up adherence.

(vi) It will be possible to enhance the treatment adherence through home visits or reminder letters to
the patients' families, and also words through another
improved patient will encourage the patients to keep
appointments regularly.

(vii) The collaboration with community leaders/voluntary
agency personnel and teachers nearer to the place
of residence of patients, with the clinic functioning
as a referral centre, will increase treatment adherence and follow-up.

(viii) Increased frequency of appointment, especially at the
beginning of a treatment regimen, providing the
opportunity for direct monitoring or supervision of
the patients may increase the follow- up.

(ix) Transport facilities and travel concessions could be
provided to the family members accompanying
psychiatric patients for follow-up.

(x) Easy accessibility of health care centres and availability of mental health care professional for immediate intervention would enhance the follow-up.

Questions

1. Define Rehabilitation.

2. What are the levels of prevention in psychiatric health
care services?

3. Identify the basic principles of psychiatric rehabilitation.

4. List down the psychiatric rehabilitation approaches.

5. Highlight the problems of rehabilitating mentally
restored people in the community.

6. What are the process involved in rehabilitation of psychiatric patient?

7. Identify the approaches that nurses can use to make the family to accept cured psychiatric patients.

8. Define vocational rehabilitation.

9. What is the role of I.L.O. in vocational rehabilitation?

10. Discuss the principles of vocational rehabilitation.

11. Explain the four means through which psychiatric patients can be reemployed.

12. Enumerate the importance of follow-up in psychiatric treatment.

13. Outline the common problems of patient's family in follow-up treatment.

14. How will you improve the treatment adherence and follow-up of psychiatric patients? Give your suggestions.

———

THE ROLE OF THE NURSES

The role of the nurses in hospital and community in psychiatric nursing

I. Nurse's role in mental hospitals

Early the role of nurses in mental hospital was characterised by custodial care, which ranged from humanistic to neglectful and cruel. Frequent baths, a wholesome diet, and "suitable exhilaration" of the mind were the primary modes of treatment for the depressed patient. The more severely disturbed were also provided these forms of therapy but were restrained in their beds to prevent them from injuring themselves or others.

The nurse's role was primarily to oversee patient care and to ensure smooth ward operation. House keeping, dietary management and laundry care commonly became the nurse's responsibility. Thus, the early nurse was the manager of a ward than a provider of direct patient care.

The reforms of the nineteenth century had great impact on hospitalised patient psychiatric nursing. The care of patients stressed humane approach, and the scientific understanding of the causes and treatment of mental illness was of primary concern. Nurses became key figures in milieu therapy and therapeutic communities.

Nurses participated actively in physical therapy, chemotherapy, psychosocial therapy and behaviour therapy. Her role was well-acknowledged in various therapeutic approaches of psychiatric patients, either individually or in psychiatric team.

Nurse's role in multi–disciplinary team

The psychiatric team consists of psychiatrist, clinical psychologist, psychiatric social worker and psychiatric nurse. The purpose of this team is to provide a forum in which these members democratically share professional knowledge and together evolve a therapeutic plan of action. It implies that psychiatric nurse has an equal opportunity to share what she has learned about the patient, and her contributions are welcomed in developing a definite goal-directed plan of action.

To function as an equal member in the multi-disciplinary team, she needed academic and professional back ground equivalent to that of her colleagues. Nursing educators implemented changes in curriculum and included psycho dynamics and interpersonal theory, communication skills, and skills in understanding and working with other disciplines.

Nurse's role in nursing process

If anything is unique to nursing, it is the nursing process. It is an "interactive" problem-solving process used by the nurse as a systematic and individualised way to fulfill the goal of nursing care.

Today's in-patient psychiatric nurse use the nursing process to provide care to individuals, families and groups. The purpose of nursing process is to maximise a patient's positive interactions with his environment, his level of wellness and his degree of self–actualisation. The nursing process enhances helping, interpersonal relationship; the nurse interacts with a patient to analyse and meet his bio-psychosocial needs.

Nurse's role in dependent, interdependent and independent functions

The most familiar dependent nursing functions involve carrying out the physician's orders. The nurse is responsible for giving treatments and medications accurately and on time. The nurse assures that the patient receives all the prescribed laboratory tests, psychological tests and other appropriate consultations.

The nurses interdependent functions may range from sharing information with the health team to acting as co–therapist with members of other disciplines in family or group therapy.

Independent nursing functions often give rise to greatest sense of job satisfaction. These functions can range from taking vital signs to carrying out special types of nursing observations and supervision. Together the nurse a id the patient develop goals and determine the course that seems most likely to lead to accomplishing these goals. Along the way the nurse must decide what teaching is necessary for the patient, his family and significant others. The nurse must judge how much can be learned from the patient's milieu and what needs must be met within the patient's home environment, community or employment situation. Nurse also provides vital link in bridging the gap between in-patient hospitalisation and successful reintegration into the community.

Nurse's role in patient's involvement

Nurses encourage the patients to take active participation in identifying their health needs, solutions to solve problems, and also meeting the health needs and solving their own problems. Nursing rounds are one method of encouraging the patient to participate. The patient is interviewed by a senior nurse in front of members of the nursing staff who are working directly with him. The patient is encouraged to discuss both useful and non-productive experiences in his hospitalisation. The patient is asked how he believes the nursing staff can best help him reach his goals. He is urged to identify his internal and external resources and to capitalise on these strengths during his hospitalisation and when he returns to the community.

Psychiatric nurse's role as a primary nurse

Primary nursing is characterised by the assignment of one nurse to coordinate the total nursing care of a patient, from admission to discharge. This provides highly individualised, comprehensive care with a degree of continuity that other nursing care delivery models cannot provide. The assumption of 24-hour responsibility sets the primary nurse apart from other nurses. The primary nurse assesses the patient's nursing needs, develops an around–the–clock plan of care and evaluates the results. Primary nurses may delegate the responsibility of implementing the care plan, but they are accountable for providing written and verbal directions.

Primary nurse has three basic characteristics – autonomy, authority and accountability. Primary nurse with autonomy collaborates with other disciplines. Other health professionals are used by the primary nurse as resources and consultants. However, the nursing care plan is developed by the primary nurse and the patient. Primary nurses must have the authority to develop and implement a total comprehensive nursing care plan on a 24-hour basis. She also needs to stand accountable for all of her decisions and actions.

By incorporating the concept of primary nursing in an in-patient psychiatric setting further strengthens the one-to-one relationship between the patient and the nurse, and that itself becomes nursing therapy.

Nurse's role in mental health education to patients

Nurses develop intimate contact with the psychiatric patients. Each opportunity of interaction with patients are utilised to give formal and informal patient education. The education process begins with the orientation of the patient and the significant others to the hospital. Policies, procedures and therapeutic activities are explained. She gives psycho-education explaining the nature of psychiatric illness that patient has, its treatment course and the expected prognosis to patient and his family.

Nurse conducts group education programme to give community living skills, communication skills, resocialisation skills, and assertiveness training.

Nurse's role in milieu therapy

Milieu therapy is a "scientific manipulation of the environment aimed at producing changes in the personality of the patient ". The word "milieu" was first used to mean a scientifically planned environment by Bettleheim and Sylvester in the late 1930's and early 1940's.

Milieu therapy provides the minutely detailed interpersonal environments based on the psychodynamic needs of a "carefully diagnosed" patient. Environmental manipulation based on patients need can itself be the primary treatment as well as a supporting or complementary aspect to other forms of treatment.

Psychiatric nurse makes use of milieu therapy in 3 different ways, namely:

(i) Patient's strengths are optimally used by the scientific manipulation of the institutional environment.

(ii) Patient's abilities are constructively made to influence their own treatment, the treatment of others and to some degree the organisational structure of the hospital.

(iii) Pervasive, therapeutic staff involvement is used for the successful treatment of seriously disturbed patients.

Psychiatric nurse is the whole sole person in this environment therapy. She manipulates the environment with less stimuli as calm and quiet to suit manic patients, keeps environment free from all sharp instruments and safe for high suicidal risk patients, prepares the environment with high provoking stimuli to depressive patients, etc. Since the patient's environmental interaction has a therapeutic effect, the environment is manipulated for the treatment purpose.

232

Nurse's role in therapeutic community

According to Kraft, "the therapeutic community is a very special kind of milieu therapy in which the total social structure of the treatment unit is involved as part of the helping process". All social and interpersonal interactions in the hospital are the main therapeutic tools used to bring about specific changes in the patient. Whereas in milieu therapy the emphasis is on the manipulation of the environment to bring about changes in the patient's behaviour.

Maxwell Jones (1959) was the person who originated the concept of therapeutic community. Accordingly, the total resources of the staff, the patient, their relatives, and the institution are pooled for the purpose of treatment. Nurses must encourage patient's active participation in his care planning.

Salient features of therapeutic community are:

(i)   Free communication both within and between staff and patient group.

(ii) Communications are directed towards the modification of patient's attitude, behaviour and role performance.

(iii) Atmosphere in the community will be democratic as opposed to hierarchial; rehabilitative rather than custodial, permissive instead of limited and controlled.

(iv) Nurses will be more communal with the patient instead of displaying all the time therapeutic role.

(v)   Environment will be essentially permissive and flexible.

(vi) Patient's activities are individualised and the role

of patients are unspecified and their participation is completely voluntary.

(vii) A compulsory daily community meeting that all staff members have to attend and all patients are encouraged to attend.

(viii) Group responsibility is emphasised and opportunities for corrective learning experience is deliberately provided.

(ix) The primary role of staff is to help the patients gain new insights and test new behavioural patterns.

(x) Problems of the patients are discussed and the solutions are sought in the small group therapy sessions following each community meeting.

(xi) Patient government or ward council is to deal with practical unit details such as privileges and house keeping rosters. Staff member is available to the patient government, and all decisions are fed back to the community through the community meetings.

(xii) Staff meeting or review is essential to on-the-ward training. It gives opportunities for the staff members to examine their own responses, expectations and prejudices.

(xiii) Living-learning opportunities are provided to the patient within the social milieu. Thus, the therapeutic community is like a "school for living" in which the patient learn to meet the demands of everyday life.

(xiv) Feed back is one of the fundamental concepts in therapeutic community practice.

Other activities in therapeutic community

Work groups, admission meetings, badminton groups and pottery groups are some of the creative activities included in therapeutic community. In addition, individual reviews, encounter groups, projective art sessions, occupational therapy workshop sessions, and patient meetings are found. Three other groups also have been created for this particular community. The "leavers group" is designed to look at the feelings and problems related to leaving the community. In this group the need for further treatment is discussed. The "concern group" is composed of patients who would clarify the aim and purpose of the hospital and the individual's role in it. "The Committee" is composed of five patients, one from each small psychotherapy group and a number of staff members. It functions as a feedback source to the community meetings and to the patient's meetings.

Nurse's role in chemo, psycho, socio and physical therapies

As earlier discussed, nurses play interdependent role. They prepare patients for therapy and assist the therapist to administer therapies. Nurses take care of the patients after the therapics and intervene in the nursing problems appropriately. Nurse's role in chemo-therapy, especially in identifying the sideeffects and reporting it to doctors and intervening the patients in time are considered vital. Similarly post-ECT patients also require assistance from nurses to overcome with sideeffects of ECT. In psychosocial therapy, nurses take independent therapist's role to provide various activity therapies like dance therapy, horticultural therapy, bibliotherapy, etc.

Day-to-day activities of a nurse in the mental hospital

Nurse's functions and responsibilities can be categorised into:

1. Patient care
2. Education and supervision
3. Ward management
4. Interpersonal relationships and communi cation.

1. Patient care

(i) Assess patient's needs

(ii) Give individualised nursing care according to their needs.

(iii) Develop care plans to meet the long-term goals.

(iv) Provide facilities to meet personal hygiene for those who can do by themselves.

(v) Assist multidisciplines in diagnosing and in thera-peutic measures. For example, giving tokens for desirable behaviour.

(vi) Provide therapeutic environment.

(vii) Distribute food to patients and feed those who are unable to feed themselves.

(viii) Observe, do mental status exam, report and record.

(ix) Set limit for patient's behaviour.

(x) Provide activities to channelise patient's energy with constructive work as a source of bringing out their personality. It increases their self-esteem.

2. Education and supervision

(i)   Supervises the work of subordinates, and changes the misconception and negative attitudes of class D officials and the family members of patients towards mental illness through health education.

(ii)   Finds opportunity to give group and individual mental health education.

(iii)   Helps the nursing students to learn psychiatric nursing and assists them to dentify mental mechanisms used by patients.

3. Ward management

(i)   Writes daily report of acutely ill patients.

(ii)   Reevaluates the chronic patient's progress once in a week and records it.

(iii)   Assesses the cleanliness of the ward and takes steps to improve it.

        For instance, slippery watery floor would cause fracture to manic running around patients; open loose hanging wire would tempt the suicidal ideas in patients, etc.

(iv)   Hands over and takes over patients, briefing with emphasis on the behavioural changes that are seen in them and the kind of attitude shown to them. It helps every shift nurses to be consistent with their approaches to patients.

(v)   Accompanies multidisciplinary team for clinical rounds and gives report based on her observations.

4. Interpersonal relationships and communication

(i) Establishes relationship with patients, their families and with team members.

(ii) Coordinates the nursing services with psycho-social therapies.

(iii) Communicates the patient behaviour that requires emergency attention to the concerned people. For example, an escape of patient from mental hospital is intimated to the police, unit consultants and to family.

(iv) Keeps link between patients, their families and with the treating team.

(v) Shares the knowledge about community resources with patients and families for future rehabilitation.

II Role of a nurse ir community psychiatric nursing

Community mental health is best defined as "all activities undertaken in the community in the name of mental health".

The basic model of community mental health was defined by Gerald Caplan in 1967. The predominant characteristics of community psychiatry are :

(i) Responsibility to a population for mental health care delivery.

(ii) Treatment close to the patient in community-based centres.

(iii) Provision of comprehensive services.

(iv) Multi-disciplinary team approach.

(v) Providing continuity of care.

(vi) Emphasis on prevention as well as treatment.

(vii) Avoidance of unnecessary hospitalisation.

Preventive psychiatry

Caplan discussed three levels of preventive intervention from the public health model to mental illness and emotional disturbance.

1. Primary prevention

It is concerned with reduction of incidence of new cases of mental disorders in the population by combating harmful forces that operate in the community and by strengthening the capacity of people to withstand stress.

2. Secondary prevention

It involves reducing the prevalence of a disorder by reducing its duration. The activities included in this prevention are early case finding, screening and prompt effective treatment.

3. Tertiary prevention

It attempts to reduce the severity of a disorder and associated disability.

Nurse's role in primary prevention

The primary prevention has a vital role of ascertaining the at-risk population and high-risk situations wherein stressful life events are the precipitating factors.

The nurses could play a major role in identifying high-risk groups and prevent the occurance of mental illness in them. Some of them are as follows :

(i) Antenatal care to mother, and educating her regarding the adverse effects of irradiation, certain drugs and prematurity.

(ii) Ensuring timely, efficient, obstetrical assistance to guard against the ill-effects of anoxia and injury to new born at birth.

(iii) Providing dietary corrections to those infants suffering from metabolic disorders.

(iv) Correction of endocrinal disorders.

(v) Training programmes for mentally and physically handicapped children like blind, deaf and mute.

(vi) Rendering crisis counselling to the parents of physically and mentally handicapped children.

(vii) Identifying the problems of scholastic performance and emotional disturbances among school going children and giving timely intervention. School teachers could be taught to recognise the beginning symptoms of problem.

(viii) Ensuring harmonious relationship among the members of the family, and teaching healthy adaptive techniques at the time of stress producing events.

(ix) Extending mental health education services at child guidance clinic regarding healthy child rearing practice; at parent-teachers' associations regarding the 'triad relationship' between teacher, child and parent; and at various extra-mural health agencies regarding integration of mental health into general health practice.

(x) Providing counselling services to adolescents and retired persons to pass through transitional crisis; to the members of bereavement family to accept the loss.

(xi Corrective suggestions and guidance to the culturally deprived groups to secure bio-psycho-social supplies (food, love, shelter, clothing, health, recreation, etc.) Otherwise the deprivation of it leads to alcoholism, crime and mental illnesses.

(xii) Strengthening the social support of frustrated aged and helping them to retain their usefulness.

Nurse's role in secondary prevention

The salient features of secondary prevention includes:

(i) Early diagnosis and case finding.

(ii) Early referral

(iii) Screening programmes

(v) Early and effective treatment for patient and, if necessary, to relevant family members

(v) Mental health education

(vi) Crisis intervention

(vii) Consultation services

Nurse's role in tertiary prevention

The nurses are mainly involved in rehabilitation services and follow-up services of the mentally restored. It needs long-term services.

The type of psychiatric rehabilitation services needed and to be rendered were dealt in detail in the previous unit. Some of the activities of nurses could be summarised as follows :

(i)   Social reintegration of discharged chronic mentally ill back into the community.

(ii) Finding vocational rehabilitation and job placement for the mentally restored for self-dependency.

(iii) Re-equipping the mentally restored with daily living care abilities.

(iv) Extending psychiatric rehabilitation and administration of medication at the door step of the mentally ill.

(v) Utilising the resources of the family and community for the long-term rehabilitation of mentally restored.

Nurses are unique in their ability to bridge the gap between the hospital and the community, between the psychiatrist and the community care given, and between the public and other health care providers. Therefore, nurse's role in community support service is primary.

III National mental health programme in India

1.   India is a signatory state to the Alma Ata Declaration which envisages "Health for all by the year 2000 A.D" as the goal. Efforts to ensure the achievement of this goal will have to include approaches & strategies for the improvement of all aspects of health – physical, mental & social. While the Government of India is fully seized with the formulation of a national health policy, since mental health forms an integral part of total health, a plan of action aiming at the mental health component of the national health programme needs to be put forward.

One of the very significant milestones in the organisation of primary health care (PHC) throughout the world is the Alma Ata Conference organised by the World Health Organisation in 1978. This forum provided an opportunity to examine the issues in PHC and develop an international commitment to the concept. It recommended that the PHC should include at least:

"Education concerning prevailing health problems, and the methods of identifying, preventing and controlling them, promotion of food supply and nutrition, adequate supply of safe water, basic sanitation, maternal and child health care including family planning, immunization against major infectious diseases, prevention and control of locally endemic diseases, appropriate treatment of common diseases, and injuries, promotion of mental health and provision of essential drugs".

It is to be noted that promotion of mental health forms one of the eight components of PHC. Although mental health promotion is listed last but it is not the least programme.

2. Primary mental health care

It includes removing misconception about mental illness, preventing the occurrence of mental illness, make early diagnosis and give early treatment to mentally ill, and rehabilitate the mentally ill with available resources within himself and in the community.

3. Importance of mental health care services through PHC

An analysis of the present situation in the area of needs, services and facilities available in mental health field, will make one realise how important it is to introduce mental health care services through the existing system of primary health care in the country.

i) Magnitude of the problem/emphasis the need

According to most of the survey about 10-20 per 1000 of the population are affected by a serious mental disorder at any point in time.

Approximately, this would constitute about 10 millions (one crore) citizens of India.

The patient population, logically speaking, is distributed in urban and rural areas in the proportion of 1:3.

The figures for neuroses and psychosomatic disorders are about 2 to 3 times higher.

Approximately 20-30 million people may require our attention.

Mental retardation (slow learners) is estimated at 0.5 to 1.0 % of all children.

When other age groups are included, mental retardation would be prevalent in the range of 2 to 3% in the general population.

The number of new cases of serious mental disorders which become manifest each year (incidence) can be estimated to be roughly 35 per 1,00,000

or

about 2,50,000 new patients every year in India.

Psychiatric disturbances in children is in the order of 1 to 2%.

There is good evidence to say that about 15-20% of all patients who seek help in general health services have emotional and psychosocial problems.

ii) **Existing mental health services**

 - 48 mental hospitals have 20,000 beds.

 - 2000-3000 psychiatric beds in general and teaching hospitals, that is, one psychiatric bed per 32,500 population.

 - One half of these beds are occupied by long stay patients.

iii) **Manpower**

1500-2000	Psychiatrists
400-500	Psychologists
200-300	Psychiatric social workers
700-800	Psychiatric nurses

Majority of them are concentrated in the urban ares. From the available data it is safe to conclude that not more than 10% of those requiring urgent mental health care are receiving the needed help with the existing services.

With the methods for treatment and prevention available in modern health care, chronicity and disability can be avoided in about 80% of the cases. Complete and lasting recovery is possible in no less than 60%.

Considering the above facts, the responsibilities of mental health professionals become more evident in primary health care services.

IV. Strategies for action

In view of the gross discrepancies between needs and available services, there are essentially two approaches for immediate action.

The first approach – To direct available resources to the establishment and strengthening of Psychiatric Units in all district hospitals.

These units should become a focus of an expanding mental health service through setting up out-patient clinics and mobile teams.

In general term, the approach would be directed from centre to the periphery.

The second is – to train an increasing number of different categories of health personnel in basic psychiatric and mental health skills. There would thus be a functional infrastructure before completing, in all instances, a physical independent mental health infrastructure.

The approach would basically be directed from the periphery to the centre.

These two strategies/approaches are complimentary. Both will allow a private sector of mental health care to continue, but in the second option the emphasis of the public sector will be primarily directed towards the poor and the underprivileged. The programme when in action will directly benefit at least 200 million population living in the backward areas of the country.

V. Aims and objectives of primary mental health care services

A. Aims

1. Prevention and treatment of mental and neurological disorders and their associated disabilities.

2. Use of mental health technology to improve general services.

3. Application of mental health principles in total national development to improve quality of life.

B. Based on these aims, the following objectives can be thought of

1. To ensure availability and accessibility of minimum mental health care for all in the foreseeable future, particularly to the most vulnerable and under privileged sections of population.

2. To encourage application of mental health knowledge in general health care and in social development.

3. To promote community participation in the mental health service development and to stimulate efforts towards self-help in the community.

VI Approaches to the attainment of programme objectives

In order to achieve the objectives formulated above, the programme will adopt the following approaches:-

1. **Diffusion of mental health skills to the periphery**

This would mean that the mental health care will be spread over the existing network of services, with the aim to incorporate mental health awareness and skills at all levels of health care. Specifically, this calls for reaching the periphery (i.e. the primary health care structure at the community level, like the primary health centre, sub-centre and village health worker) in the performance of specific, relatively simple tasks. Mental health care thus must start at the gross root level.

2. **Appropriate appointment of tasks in mental health care**

The tasks to be performed at each level (village worker, sub-centre, primary health centre, district hospital, regional hospital) will be specified and a referral system set up, so that the total system works in an integrated fashion.

The community health volunteer at the village level (approximately 1 worker for 1000 population) would be expected to act as the liaison person between mental health care system and the community.

He will participate in identification and referral of patients, and will help to supervise follow-up of patients in need of long-term maintenance therapy. The multi-purpose worker (M.P.W – one for a population of 5000) who is the first-level, full-time health personnel of our health service structure would act as the first link with health service system by providing first-aid care and follow-up service.

The senior and more experienced primary health care personnel, i.e. health supervisors (health inspectors, lady health visitors, etc.) would be entrusted with the task of early recognition and management of priority psychiatric conditions which he/she would carry out under the supervision of the medical doctor at the primary health centre. Here we find the role of public health nurse is not spelled out by the national health policy planners.

What is emphasised here is that full-fledged community health nurse should also equip herself with the knowledge and skill of psychiatric nursing and thereby, she is able to supervise and teach her subordinates efficiently.

And then the medical doctor would have over-all responsibility of organising and supervising primary level mental health care. The referral system will operate in a way which will make it possible that mental health problems are handled effectively at the appropriate level of the health system.

3. **Equitable and balanced territorial distribution of resources**

Coverage of unserved and underserved population will receive a high priority.

4. **Integration of basic mental health care into general health services**

This will facilitate the application of mental health skills when dealing with patients without gross psychiatric disturbances, and identify psychosocial problems under the disguise of physical complaints.

5. Linking to community development

An important approach would be the involvement of state, district and block leadership in the implementation of the mental health programme and deal with social problems like alcohol and drug abuse, behaviour problems of childhood and adolescence including delinquency, and other negative and eventually avoidable side products of rapid socio-economic change. The linkage with other sectors like with housing, education, town planning and legal agencies, to enhance the total mental health care awareness as well as for the application of mental health care skills and knowledge for all persons.

6. Mental health care programme

The service component will include three sub-programmes, treatment, rehabilitation and prevention.

Treatment : Specified forms of treatment would be given based on morbidity categories. But spotting out of cases and making diagnosis would be done at different levels.

a) Primary care at the village and sub-centre level

1. Management of psychiatric emergencies through simple crisis management skills.
2. Administration and supervision of maintenance treatment for chronic psychiatric conditions.
3. Recognition and management of grandmal epilepsy.
4. Liason with local school teachers and parents for the management of children with MR and behaviour problems.

5. Counselling in problems related to alcohol and drug abuse. These tasks would be performed in accordance with MPW's manual. For each task, an appropriate difficulty/severity level will be specified, beyond which the problems would be automatically referred to the next level of health care.

b) Primary health centre level

1. Supervision of the MPW's performance of specified mental health tasks.

2. Elementary diagnostic assessment of cases, and performing a standardised basic neurological examination.

3. Treatment of functional psychosis.

4. Treatment of uncomplicated cases of psychiatric disturbances associated with physical diseases like malaria, typhoid, mild to moderately severe depressive states, anxiety syndromes and initial stages of functional psychoses with appropriate drugs.

5. Management of uncomplicated psychosocial problems.

6. Epidemiological surveillance of mental morbidity in the area and compilation of estimate of needs and plan the future programmes with modification.

7. Mental health training programme :

Only very few hospitals among 48 mental hopitals have got trained psychiatric personnel. With the existing manpower it is not possible in near future to deliver mental health care to all those who immediately require it.

251

So as an immediate solution we will have to train as large a number of health personnel of all categories as possible in the minimum essentials of mental tasks at their own level of performance as discussed now.

8. Outline of plan of action :

It onsists of set of targets and detailed activities.

Targets

a) Within one year each state of India will have adopted the present plan of action in the field of mental health.

b) Within one year the Government of India will have appointed a focal point within the Ministry of Health specifically for mental action.

c) Within one year, a National Co-ordinating Group will be formed comprising representatives of all states, senior health administrators, and professionals from psychiatry, education, social welfare and related professions.

d) Within one year, a task force will have worked out the outlines of a curriculum of mental health for the health workers dentified in the different states as most suitable to apply basic mental health skills, and for medical officers working at PHC level.

e) Within five years, at least 5000 of the target non-medical professionals will have undergone a 2 week training on mental health care.

f) On the recommendation of a task force, appropriate psychiatric drugs to be used at

PHC level will be included in the list of essential drugs in India.

g) Psychiatric units with in-patient beds will be provided at all Medical College Hospitals in the country within 5 years.

Although there are 12 targets, the above seven targets demand immediate recognition.

Nursing educators and administrators should now start revising nursing curriculum and incorporate elements of community mental health nursing at different stages. All category of nursing personnel should be called for time to time orientation courses. In-service education programme should cater to the nurses already on job. Continuing education programme should take up mental health and psychiatric nursing theme in organising the programmes.

Mental health nursing researchers would raise adequate data regarding the "assets and liabilities" of mental health problems of the community. Action-oriented researches to be conducted to develop the appropriate nursing modalities to meet the diverse needs of the community.

Questions

1. What is the role of nurses in psychiatric hospital?

2. Write short notes on :

   i) Nurse's role in multi disciplinary team.

   ii) Primary nursing in psychiatric setup.

   iii) Milieu therapy.

iv) Nurse's role in therapeutic community.

v) Job description of nurses in psychiatric ward.

3. What is the role of a nurse in community psychiatric nursing?

4. What is NMHP? Discuss the salient features of NMHP.

5. Write short notes on :

i) Nurse's role in primary prevention of psychiatric care.

ii) Secondary prevention and nurse's role.

iii) Psychiatric nursing in tertiary prevention.

iv) Existing mental health services in India.

ATTITUDE TO MENTAL ILLNESS

Adaptation required in meeting basic and nursing needs

Each individual is unique and has his own potential for growth. A nurse who believes this, can assume a positive attitude towards each individual. She will be able to look at the strengths and assets of the individual rather than looking at only his weaknesses and problems. The aim should be to achieve the maximum potential without being discouraged by his deficiencies.

Common attitudes needed to be used in psychiatric nursing are:

(i) Permissiveness (Indulgence or non-judgement)

This attitude allows and encourages any evidence of initiation on the part of the patient; he is encouraged to express his wishes and make his own decisions whenever possible. The nurse accepts his behaviour. The nurse allows deviations (minor) from the ward rules but permissiveness is never allowed to encroach upon the safety and peace of the group. Such attitude can be a problem in a group setting, so it has to be used very judiciously.

This attitude is indicated for patients who are subjected to denial of self-expression and patients who are afraid of reality.

(ii) Reassurance

The nurse is expected to use every possible way to reassure the patient, which may vary from the tone of the voice to actual protection from teasing, threat or annoyance from other patients. She may reassure by verbal reassurance or by staying with him.

Reassurance is indicated for timid, frightened, insecure or extremely anxious patients. It is also frequently used with the newly admitted patients.

(iii) Firmness (kind firmness)

The nurse sets a limit for an acceptable behaviour. She is positive and firm in dealing, yet kind and approachable. The patient may be told that the hostile speeches in the public or his physical attacks on others are not acceptable. If it occurs, it should be dealt with promptness, firmness and kindness. Diverting the patient with a constructive work may be helpful. If physical force such as restraining is needed, it should be done for a short while with minimum discomfort to the patient. The reason for restraining has to be told to the patient. While restraining the patient, care must be taken to prevent injury to the skin necrosis of tissue and stoppage of blood circulation. After the release of restraint, it must be forgotten and patient must not be reminded of it.

Firmness is indicated for patients who are depressed and wish to harm themselves. It may also be useful for aggressive or uninhibited patients. For depressed patients, nurses may assign some menial work to do in the ward. The firmness is used to make him to adhere to this task, to bring out his hostility towards nurses and others in the form of verbal out-burst, which is therapeutic for him.

(iv) Active friendliness

This means an active interest in the immediate welfare of the patient. Accepting the patient and meeting his needs before he expresses it are the ways nurses express their genuine interest towards him. She is consistent but little flexible and informal.

This attitude is specially indicated for emotionally deprived patients, e.g. Schizophrenics.

(v) Passive friendliness

The nurse expresses her interest in the patient but waits for him to make the first advance before responding. The nurse needs to be warm, giving and sincere, never failing the patients. She accepts rebuffs without taking offence, and may need much waiting and patience until the patient shows signs of response.

This is indicated for shy patients and those who are afraid of active friendly attention.

(vi) Matter of factness

It is simple but difficult to practice. This attitude dictates that a nurse should not to be defensive but carry out her role calmly and pleasantly. This is for the patients who are always nagging, complaining or asking for sympathy, which the nurse must ignore and go about her routine yet remaining friendly towards the patients.

(vii) Watchfulness

Watchfulness is the first rule of any psychiatric hospital. But for special cases like suicide, escape or who harm others, it may be ordered specifically. It needs 24-hour vigilance. Attitude of watchfulness has to be of matter of fact, frequently inspecting patient's belongings for any articles which may help him to commit suicide, escape or harm others.

Basic needs of the patients

Physiological drives are called as biological drives or organic needs. These drives become active when the physiological balance within our body, called homeostasis, is disturbed. This happens when certain physiological needs are not being properly satisfied. When the psychiatric patients are preoccupied with their psychotic ideas and keep responding to their hallucinations, they tend to ignore these needs. It becomes the responsibility of nurses to help the patients in meeting the basic needs like nutrition, rest, sleep, personal hygiene, and eliminations etc.

Emotional needs are acquired through experiences of living and interacting with other human beings. Some of the emotional needs are:

(i) Need for acceptance

Acceptance conveys the feeling of being loved and cared. Psychiatric patients are usually ignored and neglected by their families and community. Therefore, the nurses must communicate the feelings of acceptance towards them.

(ii) Need for self-esteem

Self-esteem is the individual's personal judgement of his own worth obtained by analysing how well his behaviour conforms to his self-ideal.

Mainly the patients with depression express hopelessness, helplessness and worthlessness. Nurses must work towards increasing the self-esteem of patients.

(iii) Need for attention and recognition

Attention and recognition should be given upon each contact with the patient as it brings sense of satisfaction to the patients over their performance. Recognition of their inner strength and appreciation of their constructive behaviour reinforce the desirable behaviour in them and increase their self-esteem.

(iv) Need for feeling of security

Physical safety and the sense of psychological security are essential to keep the individual free from tension.

Most of the individuals develop anxiety features because of the sense of threat to their biological integrity or ego system. Non-puritive and non-judgemental attitude of the nurses provide the feeling of security to the patients.

(v) Need for understanding

To identity the exact nature of problem nurses need to explore information from the patients. Because of their mental illness, patients fail to bring out the covert problems. Recognising and reflecting those covert emotional problems of the patients from their verbal and non-verbal communication by nurses help them to meet their need for understanding.

(iv) Need for communication

Every individual communicates constantly from birth until death. All behaviour is communication and all communication affects behaviour. Communication is the vehicle for establishing a relationship, since it involves conveying information and exchanging thoughts and feelings. Talking helps the patients to ventilate his feelings, thereby relieves tension and anxiety.

(vii) Need for dependence

To find satisfaction in life people must be involved with positive interpersonal relationship. It gives the experience of closeness to each other. The dependency relationship enhances open communication of feelings and deep empathic understanding. When the need for dependency is not met, the individual feels lonely, which is very painful. The pain of loneliness can be shared empathically to some extent. Nurses could intervene in the patient's loneliness and meet the need of dependence with her active interpersonal relationship.

Similarly, patients also express the need for interdependency and independency. Based on the requirement, nurses could plan various group activities in the ward to meet the interdependency and independency needs of the patients.

The nurse and individual patient

There are general principles that apply to the care of all who show behaviour disorder. Everyone has certain basic needs that must be met no matter what disease he is suffering from. The principles are general which are applicable to mentally ill patients as well as physically ill, where his illness is usually associated with emotional disturbance to some degree.

These principles are based on the concept that each individual has an intrinsic worth and dignity and he has potentiality to grow.

1. Accept the patient exactly as he is

Acceptance conveys the feeling of being loved and cared. Acceptance provides the patient with an experience which is emotionally neutral, where he finds unlearning of his sick behaviour is less threatening before he can re-learn the art of living with himself and with others.

Acceptance does not mean complete permissiveness, but setting of positive behaviours to convey to him the respect as an individual human being. Acceptance is expressed in the following ways :

(i) Be non-judgemental and non-punitive

We don't judge patient's behaviour as right or wrong, good or bad. Patient is not punished for his undesired behaviour. All direct and indirect methods of punishing must be avoided.

Chaining, restraining, putting him in a separate room are some of the direct punishments. Ignoring his presence or withdrawing his importance are few ways of giving indirect punishment.

(ii) Show interest in the patient as a person

This can be demonstrated by :

a) Studying patient's behaviour pattern.

b) Making the patient aware in a subtle manner that you are interested in him.

c) Seeking out a patient.

d) Using time spent with him on those things he is interested in.

e) Being aware of his likes and dislikes.

f.) Explain when his demands cannot be met.

g) Dealing with his comments, complaints, and expression of approval realistically.

h) Accepting his fears as real to him.

i) Avoiding subjects on which he feels sensitive.

j) Listening to him.

(iii) Recognise and reflect on feelings which patient may express

The nurse acts as a sounding board for patient's strong or negative feelings. The nurse develops skill in identifying the feelings actually expressed. For example, when a patient says "I would like to break someone's neck", we understand that he is angry at somebody and is expressing the anger. "I am a dead person" (feeling of worthlessness, etc.)

When patient talks, it is not the content that is important to note, but the feeling behind the conversation is more important. That has to be recognised and reflected.

(iv) Talk with a purpose

Nurse's conversation with a patient must revolve around his needs, wants and interests. Nurse's responses must guide her patient. Indirect approaches like reflection, open-end question, focusing on a point, presenting reality are more effective when the problems are not obvious.

Avoid evaluative, hostile, probing responses and use the understanding responses which may help the patient to explore his feelings.

(v) Listen

Listening is an active process. Two ears are required for what the patient says verbally and the 'third ear' is required for what patient is otherwise nonverbally saying.

Encourage patient to talk through brief, non-directive comments showing interest in what patient is saying.

(vi) Permit patient to express strongly-held feelings

Strong emotions bottled up are potentially explosive and dangerous. It is better to permit the patient to express his strong feelings without disapproval or punishment. Feelings of anxiety, fear, hostility, hatred or anger should be expected, tolerated and allowed to express. Expression of these negative feelings may be encouraged in verbal or symbolic manner. The nurse must accept the expression of patient's strong negative feelings quietly and calmly. In other words a nurse makes the patient as comfortable with his illness as possible.

2. Use self-understanding as a therapeutic tool

Self-understanding leads to understanding of others. Knowing how one ought to feel or act is not important but to understand why one behaves the way she does is vital. Patient's behaviour can produce lot of anxiety or fear in the nurse, and she ought to understand why she is anxious or frightened.

We can understand ourselves better by

(a) Exchanging personal experience freely and frankly with our colleagues, or by

(b) Discussing our personal reaction with an ex perienced person, or by

(c) Participating in group conference regarding our patient care, or by

(d) Introspecting on why we feel or act the way we do.

3. Use consistent behaviour to increase patient's emotional security

Consistency in our approach is needed to develop a feeling in patient that he can depend on the people working in the ward. Our consistency must reflect in our attitudes, ward routine and defining the limitation placed on the patient. Consistency could be demonstrated by :

(a) Patient to be constantly and continuously exposed to an atmosphere of quiet acceptance.

(b) Consistency to be maintained from nurse to nurse and shift to shift which must be planned properly.

(c) Permissiveness to be limited, e.g. with homicidal, suicidal, hyperactive and suspicious patients.

(d) Patient is allowed to feel as he does but limitations are put on his behaviour.

(e) Limit and its reinforcement requires great deal of tact and understanding and should be done in quiet and matter of fact way.

(f) Attempt to win patient's liking (favouritism) is most disastrous for the patient.

4. Give reassurance to patients in subtle and acceptable manner

Reassurance is building patient's confidence or r estoring his confidence. To give reassurance, we need to understand the meaning of experience to the patient. We need to analyse the situation as to how it appears to the patient.

While giving reassurance, we must avoid saying to the patient, statements like "you will get well", "your fears are groundless", " you are a nice person", "nothing to worry", and making false promises.

Reassurance can be given in the following manner :

(a) Be truly interested in patient's problem.

(b) Pay attention to the matters that are impor tant to the patient – a matter however in significant it may be.

(c) Allow him to be as sick as he needs to be.

265

(d) Be aware and accept how the patient really feels.

(e) Do things for the patient without asking any thing of the patient in return such as im proved behaviour or show of appreciation.

(f) Sit beside patient even when he does not want to talk. Accepting patient's silence and the physical presence of nurse can be very reassuring to the patient.

(g) Listen to personal problem without show ing surprise or disapproval.

(h) Agree that patient has a problem and think along with him to solve them.

(i) Provide patient with acceptable outlets of anxiety.

5. Change patient's behaviour through emotional experience and not by rational interpretation

Major focus in psychiatry is on feeling aspect and not on intellectual aspect. Telling and advising patients is not effective in changing behaviour.

Role play, socio-drama and transactional analysis are few ways of creating emotional experience in a patient about his own behaviour. When an alcoholic patient is told that his drunkard behaviour is more hurting to his wife, to his children and takes away his time and money, he does not agree to our interpretation. But the same is acted out by giving him a role of wife or child or an alcoholic, he gains more understanding about his troublesome behaviour.

Corrective emotional experience can bring about behaviour change. Help the patient feel emotionally secure to enable him to develop and use understanding of his own behaviour. Understanding cannot be forced, as insight and understanding of one's own behaviour is painful. Interpretation is only done when patient is ready for it i.e., secure enough to tolerate it and able to apply it to alter his behaviour. Attitudes are also not identified for the patient. When he is ready to tolerate he will identify them himself.

6. Avoid unnecessary increase in patient's anxiety

Anxiety is a feeling of fear for an unknown object or event. It is also a feeling of apprehension. It is also a threat to biological integrity or self-system (ego) of the person.

Psychiatric patients already have some amount of anxiety owing to their illness, social disapproval and seclusion from the family. Psychiatric nurses must not further increase anxiety of the patients by :

(i) Contradicting his psychotic ideas.

(ii) Demanding the patients to complete the set tasks which he cannot obviously meet.

(iii) Making him to face repeated failure.

(iv) Using big sentences, professional terms while talking to him.

(v) Careless conversation within patient's hearing about his personal life.

(vi) Calling attention to patient's defects.

(vii) Being insincere.

(viii) Giving no orientation about the wards, about his co-patients, about ward staff, policies, routines and procedure.

(ix) Threats, passing sharp commands and showing indifference.

(x) Asking questions about family, work, friends, and home which is not good for the first phase of patient-nurse relationship.

(xi) Showing nurse's own anxiety.

7. Demonstrate objective observation to understand and interpret the meaning of patient's behaviour

We need to observe what a patient says or does. Those observations need to be analysed by us to draw motivation or purpose behind his talk or action.

We improve our skills of observation by continuously predicting a patient's behaviour.

While working with a patient, learning his basic problems and then guess what he will do. If your prediction is right, ask yourself why? If the prediction is wrong again ask yourself why? Keep asking yourself what is the goal of the patient and why did he behave the way he did. While examining yourself, be objective.

Objectivity is an ability to evaluate exactly what patient wants to say and not mix up your own feelings, opinion or judgement.

Objectivity is not coldness, indifference and absence of feeling but it is an ability not to let your own judgement get confused with emotional warmth.

To be objective, you keep indulging in introspection, make sure that your own emotional needs don't take a precedence over patient's needs. Maintain an objective attitude and live a balanced life.

The indications of lack of objectivity in nurse's observations are :

(i)   Nurse is critical of the patient.

(ii) Defending or justifying herself.

(iii) Demanding that the patient should treat her in a certain way.

(iv) Evaluating the patient's behaviour right or wrong.

Nurse needs to be honest with herself. This honesty can be painful but essential.

Ability to accept the faults one cannot change, and personal limitation within herself are as important as per ability to accept her patient.

8. Maintain realistic nurse-patient relationship

Realistic or professional relationship focuses upon the personal and emotional needs of the patients and not on nurse's needs. Such a relationship is therapeutically oriented and planned, and is always based on patient's needs. Nurse's goal is not shared by the patient, neither does she seek patient's approval.

Nurse keeps analysing the interaction between himself and the patient to prepare herself to guide the patient towards mature behaviour. Nurse differentiates between patient's demands and actual needs.

Nurse-patient relationship is an interpersonal process. It is for the purpose of bringing adaptiveness, integration and more maturity in patients.

9. Avoid physical and verbal force as much as possible

Any kind of force applied on patient results in psychological trauma, unless it is a patient who needs and welcomes punishment. For example, a depressed patient welcomes the punishment or scolding as he is basically suffering from guilt of having done a mistake. Restraining the violent patient in the cot is an example of physical force. If at all this force needs to be used, the following points to be kept in mind.

(i) Carry out the procedure quickly, firmly, and efficiently with adequate help.

(ii) Do not show your anger or annoyance while tying him.

(iii) Tell him the reason of tying him and also that he will be allowed to mix with others when he has gained control of himself.

(iv) Attend to his needs as usual and never let the patient feel that he is being punished.

(v) After he has become controllable, approachable, never remind him again about the incidence.

If the nurse is an expert in predicting patient's behaviour, she can mostly prevent an onset of undesirable behaviour. Nursing team must have self-control and understanding in carrying out the procedure.

10. Provide nursing care to the patient as a person and not on control of symptoms of the disease that he has

Every behaviour is caused; understand the meaning behind the behaviour. The symptoms in him is the reflection of his problem. Two patients showing the same symptom may be expressing two different needs. For example, two patients with headache may have different meaning of the symptom to them. One may have headache beca use of sleeplessness and the other may have because of hypoglycemia. Analysis and study of symptoms are necessary to reveal their meaning and their significance to the patient.

In a psychiatric ward, for example, two patients feel hostile towards the nurse and both express it verbally. One patient having spoken may get overwhelmed by feeling of guilt and panic. The other may show a rather satisfied relief having spoken. The first patient may need help in refraining from verbal expression and help him to channelise hostility in indirect way, until she can tolerate her frank expression of hostility. The other patient may be encouraged to explore verbally, and eventually hostility of both should be understood.

11. Explain routines and procedures at patient's levels of understanding

Every patient has a right to know what is being done and why it is being done to him. Every procedure should be explained at his level of understanding

271

depending on the limitation placed on him by his symptoms. Explaining to the patient reduces anxiety. The Character of explanation depends on the patient's span of attention, level of anxiety, level of ability to decide, etc. But the explanation should never be withheld, thinking that psychiatric patients are not having contact with reality or have no ability to understand.

12. Many procedures are modified but basic prinsiples remain unaltered

In psychiatric nursing field many methods are adapted to the protective needs of the patients but the nursing principles and scientific principles remain the same.

For example, giving enema, doing surgical dressing, catheterisation and giving medication: the principles behind each remain the same, but the procedure of each treatment may be different.

The nursing principles to be kept in mind are:

(i)   Safety

(ii) Comfort

(iii) Individuality and privacy

(iv) Maintaining therapeutic affectiveness

(v)   Fine workmanship while doing procedure, and

(vi) Economy of time, energy and material.

A patient who is highly suspicious of being poisoned may refuse to have oral tablets. At that time ingestion of medication may be changed into parentral method or the same tablet may be powdered and dissolved in fruit juice and given. But the principles of nursing and scientific remain same.

Prerequisites of a psychiatric nurse

To practice as a psychiatric nurse, American Nurses Association brought out standards of psychiatric nursing in 1972 and started certifying the eligible nurses from 1973 onwards. Standards are meant for providing quality care to patients. But in India, similar one is not in existence. Hence, let us discuss what ideally are the standards and how it contributes for the better care of the patients.

American standards of psychiatric nursing in Indian context

Standard I Theory

Nurse has to apply appropriate theory that is scientifically sound as a basis for decisions regarding nursing practice.

Majority of our nurses in psychiatric setting are not adequately trained in applying appropriate theory in practice. Only a few psychiatric nurses trained at the diploma and post-graduate level in psychiatric nursing are able to provide care based on their scientific assessment.

To keep 'theory' as a prerequisite, additional training need to be given to those nurses who are already working. The present general nursing curricula revised by Indian Nursing Council in 1986, has taken care of this lacunae.

Standard II Data collection

Nurses continuously collect data that are comprehensive, accurate and systematic. Observation, interview and doing mental status examination are the few techniques used in psychiatric nursing. Acutely disturbed patients are assessed constantly. In majority of the mental hospitals, data collection does not get any special priority, but is carried out in a mechanical way.

Standard III Diagnosis

Nurses recognise the problems of the patient and name them with nursing diagnosis. It forms the basis for the next step in the nursing process. Most of the nurses need to be oriented about its importance.

Standard IV Planning

Nurses plan out the nursing actions of each patient's pooling the collective efforts of the team. For student nurses "nursing care plans" are considered as part of their learning experiences. Nurses need further motivation to practice planning.

Standard V Intervention

Nurses implement the nursing interventions independently taking assistance from their colleagues. The same gets recorded in the nurse's notes.

Psychiatric nurses are expected to implement interventions like counselling, health teaching, living- learning abilities, manipulating the environment with therapeutic goal, assisting for physical and psycho-social therapies.

Psychiatric nursing care in the Indian setting precludes the psychotherapeutic as well as psychosocial strategies by nurses. The nursing action is more often than not determined by adhoc procedures, unplanned and routine ward work.

Standard VI Evaluation

The efficacy of nursing action is evaluated. Patient's satisfaction is considered as success. Bedside rounds and clinical discussion of nurses will bring out suggestions for improving nursing approaches.

Standard VII Peer review

It is another means of evaluation to assure quality of nursing care provided for patient. Regular peer review is seen only in teaching mental hospitals. Every nurse has to actively participate to discuss the type of care given by them.

Standard VIII Continuing education

India has diploma and Masters programmes in psychiatric nursing. Nurses and the hospital authorities have to feel the need of professional and personal growth through continuing education. Organising in-service education programmes seminars, conferences, symposia and keeping well-equipped libraries are a few ways to encourage nurses towards continuing education. In many hospitals they are not available because of scarcity of funds.

Standard IX Interdisciplinary collaboration

Many of our nurses carry out only the medical instructions and invest very less time for team concept.

Different ability of team members (psychiatrists, psychologists, psychiatric social workers) could be synchronised to plan, to solve patient's problem and evaluate the services delivered.

Standard X Utilisation of community health systems

Nurses extend their service beyond the hospital boundary. They follow Caplan's model on 'preventive psychiatry' for community psychiatric nursing. She identifies the high-risk population and applies preventive measures. She also conducts mental health education programmes to remove misconception about mental illness.

Community health nurses need orientation about the integration of mental health services in the existing health care delivery system as recommended in "National Mental Health Programme in India".

Standard XI Research

Compared to U.S.A., psychiatric nursing research in India is in rudimentary state. Very few nurses publish papers. Nurses need to make use of research findings in their practice. Considering the status of nursing practice in India, it could be inferred that to reach the American psychiatric and mental health nursing standards, it requires continuous effort on the part of policy makers, nursing councils, Indian Society of Psychiatric Nurses, nurse educators, nursing administrators and nurses.

Questions

1. What are the common attitudes needed to be used by nurses towards psychiatric patients?

2. Enumerate the basic needs of psychiatric patients.

3. What are the principles of psychiatric nursing? Explain the principle of "Accept the patient exactly as he is".

4. Define standards of psychiatric nursing.

5. Discuss the possibilities of implementing standards of psychiatric nursing in India.

6. Write short notes on :

i) Nurse's attitude towards mentally ill.

ii) Basic needs of psychiatric patients.

iii) Use self-understanding as a therapeutic tool. – Discuss.

iv) Standards of psychiatric nursing.

Ways of meeting aggression and violent behaviour

Anger is a normal human emotion that is crucial for individual growth and a factor present in all relationships. When handled appropriately and expressed assertively, it is a positive, creative force leading to problem solving and productive change. When channeled inappropriately and expressed as verbal or physical aggression, it is a destructive and potentially life-threatening force.

Anger is a normal response to something a person perceives as a frustration of desires or a threat to one's needs. It is a derivation of anxiety and includes feelings of powerlessness and helplessness that may be rational or irrational. Anger may be justified or unjustified, cnscious or unconscious, intentional or unintentional.

Anger behaviours span a continuum from mild irritation and arguing, to verbally or physically abusing self or others, to uncontrollable violence. Many individuals throw things in anger, displacing their anger on objects. The repression or suppression of anger adds to the potential for verbal or physical aggression.

Definitions

Anger is an expression of the anxiety aroused by a real or perceived threat to one's rights, possessions, values or significant others.

Aggression is a forceful verbal or physical action; that is, the motor counterpart of the affect of anger, rage or hostility.

The extreme experience of anger is rage or fury. Anger can be differentiated from violence, which involves destructiveness. At this level the person is totally consumed by angry feelings and unable to control his expression. At this point violence may occur, and there is a danger to the angry person and to others who are nearby.

Violence may be defined as a behaviour that is physically assaultive and risks injury to the self, others and the environment.

Types of aggression

Aggression may be channeled externally or internally.

(i) Direct outward expression of aggression may take place through verbal or physical means.

A person may hit a wall, turn over a chair, break a window. These behaviours occur on a continuum from less severe to more severe and, as a consequence, may result in different kinds of responses to the aggressor.

(ii) Indirect, outward expression may occur through ego defense mechanisms or passive aggressive behaviour.

A person may use several defense mechanisms to deal with angry feelings. Through rationalisation, he tries to justify angry behaviour, for example, "when I get tired, I get irritated". A person may use reaction formation to disown angry feelings; while actually irritated inside about a person, he may show undue concern or an overflowing love towards him.

Therefore, a person exhibiting passive-aggressive behaviour uses passivity or submissiveness to express hostility or destructive feelings. This resistive form of behaviour is often seen as procrastination, dawdling, stubbornness, intentional inefficiency or forgetfulness.

Dynamics of aggressive and violent behaviour

Early childhood experience and acquired self organisation and direction of personality growth are important.

When an individual is exposed to the necessity for continuously struggling to achieve security and a sense of confidence, he usually over-compensates by open rebellion against the edict. Aggressive self-assertion is shown by an attempt to dominate the environment through sheer activity. The underlying tension and hostility are expressed in frantic activity, in outbursts of destructiveness, in the use of ridicule, and in rage at any restriction or obstacle.

Range of behaviour

(i)   Delusion of grandeur

(ii)   Overactive

(iii) Limited attention span

(iv)   Flight of ideas

(v)   Circumstantiality

(vi)   Vulgarity and obscenity

(vii) Teases others and acts the clown

(viii) Irritable

(ix) Rebels restrictions

(x) Neglects food, rest and elimination

(xi) Dehydration and loss of weight

(xii) Poor resistance to infection

Phases of aggressive behaviour

Smith's stress model (1981) includes the assault cycle with five stages of a predictable pattern or chain of aggressive responses to emotional or physical stress. In instances in which patients are repeatedly assaultive, it can be observed that their behaviour patterns are ritualistic, stereotypical and automatic. As the acuity of the aggressive response increases, there is a comparable decrease in the patient's problem-solving abilities, creativity and spontaneity and behavioural options.

The five-phase assault cycle adapted from Smith (1981) includes the following :

(i) **Triggering phase** : The stress-producing event occurs, resulting in a number of stress responses. These include muscular tension, changes in voice quality, signs of readiness to retaliate, tapping, pacing, repeat verbalisations, non-compliance, restlessness, irritability, suspiciousness, perspiration, tremor, glaring, a change in breathing.

(ii) **Escalation phase** : Responses represent escalating behaviours that indicate movement towards loss of control. These include a pale or flushed face, screaming, swearing, high agitation, hyper sensitivity, threats, demands, clenched fists, loss of reasoning ability, provocative behaviours.

(iii) **Crisis phase** : A period of emotional and physical crisis in which a full-blown battery (carrying out the threat of injury is defined as battery) occurs. It includes fighting, hitting, kicking, scratching, throwing things.

(iv) **Recovery phase** : A period of cooling down in which the person slows down and returns to normal responses. Behaviours may include accusations, recriminations, lowering of the voice, and change in conversation contents.

(v) **Post-crisis depression phase** : This phase includes crying, apologies, reconciliatory interactions. Repression of assaultive feelings may convert to hostility that later appears as negative actions such as passive aggression.

Nursing care

The nursing care of the patient with aggressive behaviour directed outwardly as well as inwardly, differs in the specific types of nursing problems likely to be presented.

Control of violence

A patient who loses control of his anger becomes violent. The nurse in the psychiatric setting must develop the ability to deal with violent behaviour in a way that minimises the danger.

Prevention of violence is preferable if it is possible. The intense anxiety associated with violent feelings is communicated interpersonally. By empathising and carefully observing patient's behaviour, the nurse may be able to anticipate a violent outburst. Sometimes when a patient is on the verge of losing control, the atmosphere of the nursing unit is filled with tension. When the nurse becomes aware that tension is mounting, intervention may avoid an outburst. The nurse may isolate the disturbed patient from the rest of the patient group, may talk with the patient if he is receptive to this approach, and may give prescribed medication. Some patients respond to vigorous physical activity to express their anger, but this approach should be used with care, since it may precipitate loss of control.

While speaking with the patient, nurses must speak softly, slowly and with assurance. Directions should be clear and concise. It may be useful to help the patient verbalise his feelings. The nurse should take care to protect the patient's self-esteem and dignity.

Self-protection is a concern when the nurse is working with a potentially violent patient. The nurse should never fail to take adequate precautions for her own safety. The recommended precautions are as follows:

(i)   Never see a potentially violent person alone.

(ii)   Keep a comfortable distance away from the patient. Stay at least arm's length away from the patient

(iii) Maintain a clear exit route for both the staff and patient.

(iv)   Be prepared to move; violent patients can strike out suddenly.

(v)   Be sure the patient has no weapons in his possession before approaching him.

(vi)   Search the patient for any weapon (ask the patient to keep on a table or floor rather than fighting with him to take it away).

(vii) If it is necessary to restrain a patient, have an adequate number of nursing staff on hand.

Once the decision to restrain the patient has been taken, it should be acted upon immediately. Negotiating with the patient is generally futile. A minimum of four people are necessary, one for each limb. Remember, the patients can also bite. The presence of a nurse talking to the patient while the other person restrain him often calm him and renders the patient more complaint. Once in restraints, a patient should never be left unobserved.

For restraining, leather belts, padded bandages, etc. are used. (Avoid using plain bandage, ropes, etc.).

(viii) Give prescribed anti-anxiety or antipsychotic medication when it is needed.

(ix) Be supportive to the patient and intervene to increase his self-esteem.

(x) Avoid excessive stimulation (loud voice, abusing, pointing to patient, threatening him, excessive eye contact, promise etc.)

(xi) Remove all the sharp weapons (knife, scissors, razor, etc.), open electric circuit, ropes, etc. in a room where the patient is admitted.

(xii) Keep a close watch (by an attendant) or enough security for a violent patient.

All staff members in a psychiatric setting should receive training in the prevention and management of violent behaviour. The patient who has become violent may need medication or seclusion to help him gain control.

While administering medicines, tell the patient that he is upset and nervous and some medication will calm him down. Drugs concentrated in water or juice are much more acceptable to patients than injections. Avoid pills or capsules since the absorption takes too long to exert immediate effect. Effective doses are:

- Chloropromazine 50 to 150 mg (intra-muscularly) with or without promethazine (25 to 50 mg).

- Haloperidol 5 to 10 mg (intramuscularly or intravenously) with or without promethazine. Rapid neuroleptization with Haloperidol 20mg intravenously and repeated every 20 minutes to a maximum of 120 mg per day till the violence or aggressive behaviour is controlled.

- Trifluoperazine 10 to 30 mg (intramuscularly) with or without promethazine (25-50 mg) may be repeated 8 hourly.

- Diazepam 10-40 mg (intravenously, slowly) till the patient's violent behaviour is controlled. This is the drug of choice if violent behaviour is associated with epilepsy.

Electroconvulsive therapy may be used as an emergency therapy for a patient with violent behaviour.

The last step in nursing intervention with a violent patient is to review the incident with the patient after he has achieved control. This helps the patient alleviate any guilt he might be feeling or fear that he might have harmed someone. The nurse can, in retrospect, review what happened and talk about alternatives should the patient become anxious and angry in the future.

Nursing care of patients with aggressive behaviour

1. Psychotherapeutic environment

The essence of a psychotherapeutic environment for an aggressive patient is that it be unchallenging and nonstimulating. A quietly pleasant ward in physical appearance and in psychological atmosphere is necessary. Noise should be kept to a minimum, irritation avoided at all costs, and the administration of ward routine guided by the patient's needs. Since the underlying problem of hostility must be considered, the environment should restrict as far as possible the opportunities for its expression to be disastrous. The fact that stimulation can result from such varied things as bright colours, tension in others, fatigue, noise, lack of outlet energy, and numerous other factors should be taken into account when patient care is planned, both administratively and individually.

2. Inter-personal relationships

Aggressive patients need contact with persons who can accept them as they are and who function as rather neutral but warm human buffers who accept them as people and against whom they can test themselves without retaliation or judgement. Patients must be able to express their hostility and ambivalence in a calm accepting atmosphere in which their guilt is not reinforced. The limitations placed on them by their symptoms must not be used against them.

Allow the patient to verbalise his annoyance. Don't hurt the patient for his aggressiveness. Avoid complicated ideas, and long, involved explanations and discussions. Avoid comparison of him or his behaviour with other patients. Provide adequate psychological reward. Display consistent limitation over his activities. Avoid telling your opinion about him as correct or incorrect. Give positive reinforcement to build his self-esteem. Avoid appearance of rejection while interacting with him. Avoid assigning complex activities to him. Give simple tasks which he can complete easily, comfortably and in time. The day routine should be kept limited. Permit the task to be done as an expression of his need/aggression as displacement. Support a positive feeling about himself. Divert the patient during retarded stage.

Physical needs

The maintenance of adequate nutrition for patients with aggressive behaviour is essential but may present difficulty. Frequent small feedings of easily digested foods are often necessary because metabolism is either speeded up or slowed down. Eating should be carefully supervised to ensure an adequate intake, and weight should be checked at least once weekly. Careful attention of personal likes and dislikes in regard to food and attractive servings are usually worth the effort. Fluid intake is neglected by patients, and a regular schedule for giving fluids, reinforced with easily digested calorie content, should be instituted and followed through.

Elimination is a constant problem, and every effort should be made to avoid a resort to cathartics since their administration so often presents a psychological problem. Adequate fluid intake, regular toilet schedule, and adequate diet roughage should be employed routinely.

The problem of insomnia is ever present; the active patient is too busy to sleep, and the agitated patient is too tense. Warm baths in preference to showers at bed time, allowance of adequate time to settle down, and use of as many physical measures as possible are indicated. Warm milk at bed time, the reduction of stimuli, a high pillow, back rubs and a comfortable bed are all measures of importance. Careful observation as to the actual hours of sleep should be made in order that measures may be taken to avoid exhaustion.

Personal cleanliness is the responsibility of personnel for any patient in an acute stage. The period of bathing should be utilised to promote healthy personal relationships, but special attention should also be given to care of the skin, hair, and nails and to oral hygiene. Physical condition and physical well-being are closely related to emotional responses, and the patient should be kept as physically comfortable as is possible in order to add no burden to his emotional problems. Personal appearance should be kept at the highest level possible because of its effect on the patient's self-opinion and on the response of others to him.

Aggressive patients are careless in regard to personal appearance, personal cleanliness, and physical symptoms. Therefore, careful observation in regard to symptoms of physical illness is necessary. In addition, slow healing is characteristic so that prompt and efficient attention to infections and their treatment is essential.

A loss of weight and appetite goes along with an increase in the severity of symptoms, and an increase in weight and hours of sleep often presages clinical improvement. For this reason, serious efforts to improve the general physical status of the patient are included in the general plan of treatment and their importance cannot be minimised.

4. Protection

The protective needs of aggressive patients are quite high. Exhaustion, injury to others and to self, and suicide are common enough occurances to warrant constant alertness directed towards their prevention.

Exhaustion can be produced by overactivity, agitation or tension. The physical condition of such patients should be carefully observed, and indications for intercession should be acted upon. The nurse should not be confused as to the reserves of patient energy by the degree of output. Measures to avoid exhaustion are the limitation of activity by physical or chemical means, the careful avoidance of stimulation and irritation, the maintenance of fluid and caloric intake, and elimination. Accurate observation and reporting are essential.

Injury to others may occur through the impulsive gestures of overactive and aggressive patients. Close observation and thorough knowledge of the patient's behaviour patterns are aids in preventing such injuries. Recognition of mounting tension as indicated by voice changes, muscular signs of tensions, and increasing irritation are indications to take action to avoid possible injury to others. In addition, objects that can be used for assault should be removed.

Self-injury and suicide are fairly common in aggressive patients. They sustain injury because of their impulsiveness. Alert observation, distraction and occupation of the patient in some constructive activity are usually the best preventive measures. The care of injuries presents quite a problem because of the patient's lack of ability to assist in treatment. Therefore prevention is the best measure.

5. Group relations

The overactive, aggressive patient is far from being a total loss in a group. Unless there are too many like him which can be extremely disruptive, he can be quite an asset. His values are derived from the fact that he can initiate activity, although he may not carry it through, and that he can stimulate responses from withdrawn and retarded patients that a person in an authoritarian position may not be able to do. The danger to him lies in the fact that his domineering aggressiveness may draw group reaction against him, and his sensitivity may render him quite susceptible to hurt. Also, his aggressiveness may secure for him an undue amount of time and attention from personnel, which may result in a group united against him. If these precautions are kept in mind, his entrance in groups may be promoted, and assistance may be given to him when he is in difficulty by distracting him from his course of action and by substituting another that will bring peace for the moment. For him, that is all that is necessary since he is more or less at the mercy of environmental stimulation. The association with quiet patients may also tone him down somewhat since they are not particularly stimulating. If, however, their very quietness irritate him, contact with such patients should be minimised as far as possible.

6. Convalescence

The convalescent period is one of return of responsibility to the patient for his own behaviour and destiny. It is inevitable, and with this particular group of patients it involves a calculated risk. More patients actually succeed in committing suicide during the convalescent period than during the acute period, especially overactive aggressive patients. The nurse must therefore be extremely alert and not in the least lulled into a false security by the patient's seeming normality. She must always be accessible to the patient and encourage his free discussion of any topic with her in order to have an opportunity to assess his true emotional state. She must also be very tactful about this.

It is quite customary to see the patient go through a mild swing in the opposite direction from his illness, and the nurse should expect and be prepared for it. The overactive aggressive patient often has a mildly depressed period, and may have insomnia, loss of appetite or weight, and irritability. Another signal of significance is a sudden comfortable relaxation in the midst of obvious tension. Such occurrence usually indicates that the patient has made a decision, and a decision is made under such conditions may be unwise even to the point of determination of a definite method of suicide.

Approaches to the normal should be quietly encouraged. If the patient wishes to talk about his experience, well and good. Encourage it. Do not, however, embarrass a patient by talking about his acute period unless he indicates he wishes it. Even then, no judgement should ever be passed.

If the patient presents the opportunity, encouragement should be given to him to utilise his better adjustment through continued psychotherapy. The patient should also be encouraged to recognise signs in his own behaviour that may indicate a relapse and need for a return to treatment.

Guidelines for nursing intervention of patients with aggression and violence

1. Prevent physical aggression or acting outthat can cause danger to the patient or others.

    - Build a trusted relationship with patient.

    - Be aware of factors increasing the likelihood of violent behaviour and use verbal communication and/or SOS medication to control before he becomes violent.

2. Provide a non-threatening, therapeutic environment.

    - Decrease environmental stimulation by : turning stereo or television off or lowering the volume; dimming the lights.

3. Provide an outlet for the patient's feelings. Encourage verbal expression of feelings.

    - Remain with the patient and listen.

    - Use communication techniques.

    - Engage him with some physical exercise like gym.

4. Deal safely and effectively with the patient's physical aggression or acting out.

    - Give prescribed medication/seclusion restraint orders.

- Remain calm.

- Seek for assistance while restraining the patient.

- Do not use physical restraint without sufficient reason.

- Allow the patient freely to move around (within safety limits) unless restraint is required.

- Talk to him in low, calm voice. Use simple, clear, direct speech. Repeat if necessary. Do not threaten him but state limits and expectations.

5. Provide for the patient's safety and needs while in restraints or seclusion.

- When placing the patient in restraints or seclusion, tell him what you are doing, the reason for doing. Use simple, concise language in a non-judgemental matter-of-fact manner.

- Tell him where he or she is and that he or she will be safe. Assure him that staff will check on him or her.

- Apply mechanical restraints safely; do not restrain the patient lying on his or her back, but position the patient on his or her stomach or side. Check extremities for colour, temperature and pulse distal to the restraints every two hours.

- Perform passive range of motion on restrained limbs and reposition the patient at least every two hours.

- If necessary, loosen the restraints one at a time to exercise limbs or change the patient's position.

- Assess the patient with regard to safety, effects of medications, nutrition, hydration, and excretion. Offer fluids, food, and opportunities for hygiene and elimination; assist the patient as necessary.

- Reassess the patient's need for continued seclusion or restraint.

- Reorient the patient or remind him or her of the reason for restraint if necessary. Release the patient or decrease restraint as soon as it is safe and therapeutic. Base your actions on the patient's, not the staff's need.

. Remain aware of the patient's feelings (including fear), dignity and rights.

- Record vital signs. Write nurse's note, briefing patient's behaviour and the nature of restraint/seclusion used since restraint, seclusion, assault, and so forth are situations that may indeed involve legal action.

Provide for the safety and needs of other patients.

- Do not assign or allow other patients to help in restraining a patient.

- Do not allow other patients to watch the situation. Take them to a different area and involve them in a spontaneous activity.

- Talk with other patients, especially after the

situation is resolved; allow them to ventilate their feelings.

8. Deal safely with the patient who has a weapon.

- If you are not properly trained or skilled in this area, do not attempt to intervene. Keep something (like a pillow, mattress, blanket wrapped around arm) between you and the weapon.

- If it is necessary to remove the weapon, try to kick it out of the patient's hand (never reach for a knife with your hand).

- Distract the patient momentarily to remove the weapon (throw water in the patient's face, yell)

- You may need to call outside assistance, especially if patient has a gun. When this is done, the total responsibility for decisions and action is delegated to the outside authorities present.

Questions

1. Define anger.

2. What is aggression?

3. What are the different types of aggression?

4. Discuss the dynamics of aggressive behaviour.

5. How do you explain the phases of aggressive behaviour?

6. How do you prevent violence behaviour of psychiatric patients?

7. What precautions will you take while approaching violent patient?

8. Discuss the role of chemotherapy with violent patients.

9. Explain the role of nurses in taking care of the patients with aggressive behaviour.

10. Plan a nursing care of an aggressive patient based on priority of his health needs.

Depression

As early as the fourth century B.C. depression was identified as a problem requiring treatment. Hippocrates described a syndrome that is called "melancholia". He believed that it was caused by a predominance of black bile. Subsequently, Aristotle observed the problem and proposed wine and music as therapy for melancholia. Burton wrote the anatomy of melancholia describing melancholia as a disease of the head or mind. Krapelin in 1899 introduced the term manic depressive psychosis. Greek and Roman physicians used to treat depressive states by music, drama, rest and salt water.

1. Definition

Oxford Text Book of Psychiatry defines "Depressive disorders are syndromes of depressed mood, pessimistic thinking, lack of enjoyment, reduced energy and slowness".

International Classification of Diseases-10 describes as "in depressive episodes the individual suffers from depressed mood, loss of interest and enjoyment, reduced energy leading to increased fatiguability and diminshed activity. The change of mood is relatively fixed and persists over a period of days, weeks or months. This change in mood affect the behaviour, attitude, thinking and physiological functioning".

2. Etiology

Major depressive illness is more common in women than in men. Berges estimated that about 1.5 million people are treated for unipolar illness each year in the United States. Major depression occurs in mid to late 20s of age. The occurrence of depression is positively related to the family history, and 17% of depressive patients have their history as any of their relatives suffering with depression. The worldwide prevalence of depression is between 13-20 percent of the population. It has been suggested that among African people depressive disorders are uncommon.

The cause of depression can be broadly categorised as either biological or psychological.

A. Biological theories of depression

Neurotransmitter deficiency causes depression. It gives rise to 'vegetative' symptoms, symptoms that affect sleeping and eating. Typically, such a person cannot go to sleep easily, wakes periodically during the night, or more frequently wakes early in the morning and cannot go back to sleep. Appetite is usually decreased; sometimes enough to constitute anorexia with weight loss. Patients with endogenous depression benefit greatly from antidepressant drugs.

The findings of many research studies indicate that a chemical imbalance or deficiency in the brain of certain neurotransmitters cause mental state of depression. The neurotransmitters (brain amines) are norepinephrine, serotonin and probably dopamine. Most antidepressants increase the availability of neurotransmitters.

B. Psychological (psychodynamic) theories of depression

The explanations can be categorised under three general themes; debilitating early life experiences, intra-psychic conflicts, or reactions to life events.

(i) Debilitating early life experiences

Events in one's early life can lay the foundation for adult depression. The developmental theories of Freud, Erikson and Sullivan view the early years of life as foundational to life-long mental health. Early losses, maternal inconsistency, the giving and withholding of love by the care giver and various types of abuses are all explained as causative agents for mental illness. Any early life experience that could contribute to or cause lowered self-esteem and was not dealt with effectively can be a cause for depression later in life

(ii) Intra-psychic conflict

Intra-psychic conflict refers to the conflicts people have when they have mixed emotions about some behaviour, event or situation. For instance, a boy who has been brought up to refrain from sexual activity but who also has strong urges to experience sex has a real conflict. To refrain increases sexual frustration and to engage in sexual activity may cause anxiety, guilt, and fear. Later he develops depression.

(iii) Reactions to life events

Most people view depression as a reaction to life stress. Loss is a major theme – loss of a loved one through death or divorce, loss of a job, loss of self-esteem, loss of a sense of control of self and life, loss of familiar surroundings and everything those surroundings represent, and even the loss caused by a psychotic disorder can cause depression.

3. Classification of depression

Depression are broadly classified into three groups:

(i)   According to etiology (Reactive and Endogeneous)

(ii) According to symptoms (Neurotic and Psychotic)

(iii) According to course and time of life (Uni polar and Bipolar)

(1) According to etiology

Reactive depression	Endogenous depression
• Response to external factors stressful life events	• Caused by factors within the individual.
• Symptoms seen are anxiety, irritability, phobia, early night insomnia.	• Biological functioning impaired. May or may not be related to life event. Symptoms seen are constipation, weight loss, reduced libido, early morning waking.

(ii) According to symptom

Non Psychotic or Neurotic depression

- Stressful event
- Results of unconscious dynamics
- Result long standing maladaptive personality
- Insight is well presented

- At present neurotic depression is termed as dysthymia

Psychotic depression

- Disturbance in high level of functioning memory, perception, thinking
- Loss of touch with reality

- Psychotic features, Hallucination, Delusion, and Confusion

- Impairment of social and personality functioning

- Diurnal variation of mood. Feels more sad in the morning than evening
- Early morning waking.

(iii) According to course and time of life

Unipolar depression

- Repeated episodes of depression

- Episodes last for between 3-12 months, duration

- Recovery is complete between episodes

- More common in women than men.

Bipolar depression

- Repeated episodes of mood elation and depression.

- Mania episodes usually begins suddenly

- Depression tends to be of longer duration

- Episodes of both kinds often follow stressful life events.

(iv) ICD-10 classification of depression

Three varieties mild, moderate, severe as per presence of symptoms.

4. Triad of symptoms

- Depressed mood
- Loss of interest and enjoyment.
- Reduced energy leading to increased fatiguability and diminished activity.

Other common symptoms

(i)   Reduced concentration and attention.

(ii) Reduced self-esteem and self-confidence.

(iii) ideas of guilt and unworthiness.

(iv) black and pessimistic views of the future.

(v)   ideas of acts of self-harm or suicide.

(vi) disturbed sleep.

(vii) diminished appetite.

Mild depression – At least two main and two other symptoms.

Moderate depression – Three main and four other symptoms.

Severe depression – All three main and four other symptoms with severe intensity.

5. Clinical features

(i) Affect : Depressed or sad, dejection, helplessness, gloomy, pessimistic, negative feeling about self.

(ii) Thought

Slowed and decreased concentration, obsessive ideas; in severe depression, hallucination, delusion, suicide ideas.

(iii) Physical

Weakness and fatigue

Very little energy to carry out any activity.

Digestion sluggish

Constipation, decreased libido

Excessive eating and drinking

Sleep disturbance or hyper somnia.

Anorexia and weight loss

In psychotic depression early morning waking.

(iv) Psycho-motor activity

Lethargic

Regression

Purposeless movement

Agitation, irritability in some patient.

(v) Speech

Limited.

Social interaction is decreased.

Individual regret his own life.

(vi) Diagnosis

History : Detailed history from patient, his/her spouse, family members, co-workers.

303

Mental Status Exam : Depressed mood, ideas of hopelessness, ideas of helplessness, lack of initiativeness.

6. Treatment

    (i)   Medical treatment

    (ii)   Psycho social treatment

(i) Medical treatment

a) **Hospitalisation** : The first and most critical decision the physician must take is whether to hospitalise the patient or to attempt out-patient treatment. Mild depression and moderate depression may safely be treated on an out-patient basis.

Indications for hospitalisation are,

- acute depression
- severe depression with suicidal risk
- depressed patient where the family is the cause of depression and therapy is needed. For example, family and marital therapy.

b) Antidepressant drugs

Antidepressant drugs blocks the re-uptake of the neurotransmitters therapy increases the level of neurotransmitters.

Pharmacokinetics

Antidepressant drugs are easily, rapidly absorbed and extensively metabolised in the liver. They have a long action and need to be given only once a day. Absorption is usually completed within 10 hours of oral ingestion.

Dosage is always adjusted according to the individual response.

Antidepressants drugs are classified as

Unicyclic	- Bupropein	200-450 mg
Bicyclic	- Fluoxetine (prozoc)	20-80 mg
Tricyclic	- Amitriptyline	75-300 mg
	Imipramine (Tofranil)	75-300 mg
	Surmontil	75-300 mg
	Nor-tryptyline	75-300 mg
Tetracyclic	- Maprotiline	75-225 mg

Monoamino oxidate inhibitors (MAOI)

Action : Exact mechanism is unknown. It inhibits the enzyme monoamino oxidase, which normally inhibits the activity of norepinophrine and dopamine thereby storage is increased.

Drugs are	– Phenelzine	45-50 mg
	– Isocarboxazid	10-30 mg

Other antidepressants are

Dothiepin   Trazodone

Miansenin - less toxic to the heart.

Side effects of antidepressants

Central nervous system : Drowsiness, dizziness, weakness, headache, fatigue, confusion, lethargy, memory deficits, lowered seizure threshold, insomnia, tremors, ataxia.

Cardiovascular disorders : Orthostatic hypotension, tachycardia, congestive heart failure, arrhythmias.

Dermatology : Skin rash, urticaria, erythema, petechiae, photo sensitivity.

Gastrointestinal tract : Dry mouth, constipation, nausea, vomiting, diarrhoea, abdominal cramps.

Genito-urinary tract : Urinary retention, gynaecomatia.

Haemato : Agranulocytosis, thombocytopenia.

Hepatic : Jaundice, hepatitis.

c) **Lithium**

Lithium is currently the drug of choice for treatment of bipolar mood disorder and also been used in the treatment of depression.

There is a 1-2 week lag period before any appreciable response is observed. So, for treatment of depression the usual dose range is 900-2100 mg of lithium carbonate per day. The treatment is closely monitored by repeated blood levels, as the difference between therapeutic and lethal blood levels is not very wide.

Therapeutic blood lithium level is 0.8–1.8 mEq/L

Prophylactic blood lithium level is0.6–1.2 mEq/L

More than 2.0 mEq/L blood lithium level may be associated with toxicity, while more than 2.5-3.0 mEq/L blood level may be lethal.

The common acute toxic symptoms are neurological while common chronic side effects are nephrological and endocrinal (usually hypothyroidism)

The important investigations before starting lithium therapy are complete general physical examination, CBC, EKG, urine routine examination, 24-hour urine volume, renal function tests and thyroid function tests.

Unwanted effects of lithium

A mild diuresis due to sodium excretion occurs soon after the drug is started. Other common effects include tremor of the hands, dry month, a metabollic taste, feelings of muscular weakness and fatigue.

Later effects

After the initial sodium diuresis, many patients develop poor renal concentrating ability, resulting in polyuria, polydipsia. Few patients develop diabetes insipidus syndrome. Weight gain, tremor, hypothyroidism, partial hair loss in the absence of hypothyroidism, reversible ECG changes, leucocytosis, dehydration and long-term effects of kidney are also seen.

Toxic effects

Ataxia, poor concentration of limb movements, muscle twitching, slurred speech and confusion. They constitute a serious medical emergency, for they can progress through coma and fits leading to death. If these symptoms appear, lithium must be stopped at once and a high intake of fluid provided with extra sodium chloride to stimulate an osmotic diuresis. In severe cases renal dialysis may be needed. Lithium is rapidly cleared, if renal function is normal, so that most cases either recover completely or die. However a few cases have been reported of permanent neurological damage despite heamodialysis.

Lithium crosses the placenta and causes abnormalities in the babies of mothers receiving lithium in pregnancy. Lithium is also secreted into breast milk. Therefore lithium should be avoided in the first trimester of pregnancy and bottle feeding is a wise precaution.

Other drugs

Carbamazepine

For treatment and prevention of bipolar mood disorder. Especially in those patients who are refractory to lithium. And also it is effective when EEC is abnormal. Dose range=600-1600 mg/day. (Blood level=0.4-1.2 ug/ml).

(ii) Electroconvulsive therapy

Indications for ECT in depression are :

(i)   Depression with suicidal risk

(ii)   Severe refractory depression

(iii) Delusional depression

(iv)   Depression with significant antidepressant side effects.

The response is rapid, resulting in marked improvement. Usually 6-8 ECTs are needed, given three times a week. The improvement is not sustained after stopping ECTs, so antidepressants have to be given along with ECTs, to maintain the improvement achieved. The safety of this procedure has been well established.

Psychosocial treatment

Psychosocial treatment maybe indicated as an adjunct to somatic treatment and in mild cases of depression. They are:

(a) Cognitive behaviour therapy

First initiated by Beck. The aim is to correct the depressive cognition (ideation) like hopelessness, worthlessness, helplessness and pessimistic ideas and replacing them with new cognitive and behavioural responses. Because of altered style of thinking, the individual experiences negative of self and expresses hopelessness, helplessness and negative view of the future and that leads to inactiveness, and inactiveness again leads to depressed mood. To break this cycle cognitive behaviour therapy is used.

The patient is asked to focus his attention on an object in the environment or on some puzzles. So he can concentrate his mind on puzzles. The patient is also asked to write some part of pleasurable memory. The activities of him are structured. Positive reinforcement is given after completion of scheduled work. All these techniques will help the patient to distruct his negative thought and increase his self-esteem.

(b) Psychoanalytic psychotherapy

The short-term psychoanalytic psychotherapies aim at changing the personality itself rather than just ameliorating the symptoms. The usefulness is uncertain, particularly in major depression.

(c) Group therapy

Once the patient feels comfortable then group therapy can be introduced. In group therapy negative feelings such as anxiety, anger, guilt, despair is recognised. The channel to express their feelings with emotional support from others can allow emotional growth.

Patients come in contact with group members and therapist. During group process the patients recognises their own feelings and learn to know value and goodness of oneself. Negative thinking is encountered during session. Therapist encourages patients to acknowledge and tolook at all sides of an issue and select new patterns of behaviour.

(d) Supportive therapy

The aim of therapy is to bring emotional equilibrium and to support patient ego strength and positive assets.

Various techniques are employed to support the patient. They are reassurance, ventilation, occupational therapy art, play, music, relaxation, exercise, etc.

(e) Family therapy

Apart from educating the family about the nature of illness and usefulness of somatic treatment, family therapy has not been found useful in mood disorders. Another use is to decrease intra-familial and interpersonal difficulties and to reduce or modify stressors, which may help in faster and more complete recovery. The main purpose is to ensure continuity of treatment, to ensure adequate drug compliance.

7. Nursing management

The nursing interventions used in the treatment of the depressed patient flow from appropriate development of the nursing care plan. Nurses need to mainly focus on psychotherapeutic management, the nurse-patient relationship, psychopharmacology and milieu management.

(i) Nurse-patient relationship

Depressed persons suffer from low self-esteem. The most effective approach to bolster self-esteem is to accept the patient as he is (negative attitude and all), help him focus on the positive (accomplishments, good points) provide success experiences with positive feedback, keep self-help strategies simple, and help the patient avoid embarrassing social blunders (smelly clothes, unkept appearance).

Development of a meaningful relationship in which the depressed person is valued as a human being is important to his or her sense of personal worth.

The nurse working with the depressed patient must have sincere concern for the patient and be empathetic to be effective. The nurse acknowledges the emotional pain and suffering conveyed by the patient and offers to help the patient work through the pain.

Depressed persons are typically dependent. After working with the patient, the nurse may notice that he or she (the nurse) is taking on responsibility for the depression. The nurse should reward even small decisions or independent actions of patient.

Never reinforce halfucinations, delusions, or irrational beliefs. The nurse cannot agree, or arguing seems to reinforce them.

Depressed persons tend to be angry. Encourage verbal expressions of anger that helps to decrease the 'bottled up' tension.

The nurse must help depressed person to emerge from social isolation by spending time with him (even without speaking), by providing a non-threatening one-to-one relationship, by practicing assertiveness interactions, and by being accepting of the patient.

Depressed persons can have difficulty in making even simple decisions. Initially the nurse may need to make decisions for the patient.

But it is therapeutic to provide decision-making opportunities as the patient is able to comply. When possible, the nurse helps guide the patient to appropriate decisions by using problem-solving techniques; that is, what are the options, the pro's and con's of each option, and the potential consequences of each decision.

(ii) Psychopharmacology

When patient is on tricyclic antidepressants, MAOI and lithium the side effects have to be intervened. Some of them are as follows:

Side effects   **Intervention**

Tricyclic antidepressants (TCA)

Side effects	Intervention
Dry mouth	Provide frequent mouth rinses, chewing gum.
Nasal congestion	Instill decongestants.
Urinary hesitancy	Ask patient to hear the sound of running water, provide privacy, pour warm water over perineum.
Urinary retention	Catheterise for residual fluids and encourage frequent voiding
Blurred vision	Reassurance; this symptom usually subsides; caution about driving.
Constipation	Diet with roughage, laxatives as ordered.
Ataxia, sedation	Avoid dangerous tasks; day time sedation is minimised if all TCAs are given at bed time.
Confusion	Withhold the drug and inform doctor
Orthostatic hypotension	Instruct patient to rise slowly; If patient is lying down, should sit on side of bed for 1 full minute before rising to walk.Instruct to avoid standing in one place too long and to taking hot baths or showers.
Arrhythmias, Tachycardia, Palpitations	Record vital signs, withhold drugs
Decreased sweating	Instruct patient to be cautious about strenuous activity in hot weather.

313

MAOI

Agitation, Hypomania	Withhold MAOI and inform doctor.
Blurred vision, hypotension, drymouth, constipation.	See TCA interventions.
Hypertensive crisis drugrelated to food-drug or drug-drug inter-actions	Avoid these food and combinations.

Lithium

Confusion, restlessness, sleeplessness	Withhold lithium.
Nausea	Give lithium with meals.
Thirst	Instruct patient to drink 10 to 12 glasses of water every day.
Diarrohoea	Replace electrolytes.
Weight gain	Place patient on structured diet.
Sedation, blurred vision, arrhythmias, tachycardia, palpitations, dry mouth, constipation.	See TCA interventions.

(iii) Milieu management

It is an important dimension of psychiatric nursing care for the depressed patient.

(a) The patient with low self-esteem

Encourage the patient to participate in activities, including group activities, in which he will be able to experience accomplishment and receive positive feed-back. Provide successful experiences, however small.

Provide assertiveness training. It helps them learn to take care of their needs and to express their feelings along the way so that the extremes of "doormat" and "flare-up" are avoided.

Help the patient avoid embarrassing himself through socially unacceptable appearance or behaviour. Many appearance problems are directly related to the depressed person's pre-occupation, apathy, and decreased energy level. For instance, food stains on clothes, food in one's beard, an unattended runny nose, uncombed hair, urine on trousers are all commonly seen among depressed persons who "cannot" pay attention to these hygienic concerns. Help patients to have regular bath and dress appropriately.

(b) The anorexic patient

Nursing staff must take responsibility for ensuring that the depressed patient eats. The nurse must encourage the patient to eat and may even spoon-feed him if required.

Allow patient to participate in selecting preferred foods.

Promote a proper diet, adequate fluids, and exercise. Provide small, frequent meals. Record intake.

Constipation is a side effect not only of anti depressants but also of depression itself. A diet with adequate fiber content and sufficient fluids is important

If the patient will eat food brought from home, allow him to have such food.

(c)   The withdrawn patient

Depressed patients often do not want anyone around or, at least, any one to talk to them. Keep contacts with the patient, brief but frequent. Spending time with the patient is constructive, allowing the patient to isolate himself is not. Patient may need to increase physical activity before they are able to verbalise issues. Sitting in silence during an activity is better than ruminating in isolation.

(d)   The patient with sleep disturbances

Depressed persons want to sleep, but many suffer from insomnia. Activities can be substituted for the day time sleeping. Exercise often increase energy levels. Provide a quiet, peaceful time for resting. Decrease environmental stimuli (loud conversation, bright lights) in the late evening.

Provide a night-time routine or comfort measures (back rub, tepid bath, warm milk) just before bed time. Talk with the patient only for brief period(s) during night hours to help relieve anxiety and to provide reassurance before the patient returns to bed. Do not allow the patient to sleep for long periods during the day. Use SOS medications as indicated to facilitate sleep. Limit coffee especially in the evening or at night.

(e)   Suicide

The depressed patient's needs for physical safety and health require that the nurse maintain a constant vigil for the possibility of suicide and other self-destructive behaviour. The safety measures are as follows:

316

- Observe frequently or continuously on a one-to-one basis.

- Keep the environment free from potential danger such as belts, razor blades, scissors and other sharp objects. Broken glasses of window are to be immediately replaced. Hanging open wires are to be also immediately rectified.

- Be aware of the medications that the patient is taking as there are possibilities of his hoarding dosages for future lethal ingestion. Keep the ward drugs in cupboard under lock and key.

- Search him and his belongings if the patient leaves the ward or hospital for any reason upon return.

- Keep a detailed written description of "suicidal precautions" which are imple- mented when patients are identified as suicidal.

- Patient should not be left alone even in the bathroom.

- Let the patient know that his stressful situation is acknowledged and communicate that he will receive support and help in controlling his emotions/impulses.

- Gratify dependency needs during inter- personal relationship with patient as it would reduce the level of anxiety, which, in turn, decrease the risk of suicide.

- Teach him coping skills.

- Discuss with the patient about his suicidal thoughts, suicidal plans that will probably reduce his anxiety.

- Look for suicidal clues.

- Establish a "no suicide contract".

- Explore patient's strengths.
- Promote decision making ability in him.
- Set limits on him and be firm, consistent.
- Every shift nurses must be aware of suicidal risk patients.
- Convey the feelings of acceptance and belonging.
- Promote and reinforce the feelings of being useful and needed and feelings of accomplishment.

The effectiveness of nursing care is determined by changes in the patient's maladaptive emotional responses and the effect they have on present functioning.

Questions

1. Define depression.
2. What are the etiological factors involved in depression?
3. How do you classify depression?
4. Explain psychodynamics involved in depression.
5. What are the signs and symptoms of depression?
6. Discuss the medical management of patient diagnosed as depression.
7. Explain the role of Lithium in treating a depressive patient.
8. Describe psycho-social treatment of depressive patients.
9. How will you take care of a patient who is depressed?
10. How will you prevent suicide among depressive patients?

Withdrawal and mania

Withdrawn behaviour

Withdrawn means 'drawn himself back'. Withdrawal is one of coping the mechanisms to remove oneself from a threatening situation or run away from that area. Withdrawn behaviour is described as a disruption in relatedness. This involves patient's relatedness to self, others and/ or the environment. The degree of disruption can be anywhere on a continuum from mild to severe. The patient retreats from the external world and becomes increasingly self-absorbed.

Withdrawn behaviour that is mild or transitory, such as a stunned or dazed period following trauma, is thought to be a self-protecting defense mechanism. This brief period of "emotional shock" allows the individual to rest and gather resources to cope with the trauma. Withdrawal of this nature is considered normal (in that it can be expected) and is considered healthy behaviour.

Withdrawn behaviour can become increasingly severe, however, and can interfere with the patient's ability to function.

1. Definition

Beck has defined withdrawal as "it is an adaptive or coping mechanism that involves physically pulling away from or psychologically losing interest in, an anxiety producing situation, person or stressful environment".

Withdrawn behaviour is manifested by emotional and physical distancing from the external world and resulting from a disruption in relatedness between self, others and/ or the environment.

2. Dynamics of withdrawal behaviour

The early self-organisation of withdrawn individuals is self-depreciatory, causing a marked feeling of insecurity in interpersonal relationships. Often they are from a fa...ily characterised by conflict, tension and anxiety. In an anxiety-laden home, the child has difficulty in building a self-image that gives him confidence in himself as a person with an identity of his own, in developing trust in others, and in learning techniques for relating to others that contribute to his security. As a result, the repertoire of behaviours developed by the individual and used to respond to social situations is inadequate.

Under such circumstances, strong motivational systems that cannot be expressed or accepted are dissociated from the self-system. Narcissism, or self-love, and self-preoccupation become thoroughly embedded in the personality. The person becomes extremely sensitive, and the world often becomes an unpleasant place to live. Immobilisation becomes a protective device and the self-organisation becomes more and more rigid. Since the achievement of security is the immediate goal, the intellect becomes a tool for rationalisation and fogging of reality rather than a tool for reason and adaptation to reality.

The conflict between success and the struggle necessary to achieve it continues, and withdrawal from reality follows withdrawal of emotional investment in the environment. Regression follows, and the individual sinks progressively lower towards earlier stages of experience and behaviour patterns. There may be total personality disorganisation, with autistic speech, confusion and inappropriate behaviour.

3. **Characteristics of withdrawn behaviour**

    i)   Poverty of affect : Withdrawn patient has difficulty in expressing his feelings.

    ii) Apathy or expression of feelings in a very inappropriate way, like laughing without reason.

    (iii) Ambivalence : Feeling towards others change from love and hate at the same time.

    iv) Disorders of thought process with the features losing an association, and thought block.

    v)   Hearing of voices, delusions may be present.

    vi) Regression.

    vii) Negligence of personal hygiene.

Withdrawn behaviour may be seen in chronically depressed individuals, hypochondriacal persons, inaffective disorders, alcoholism, drug addiction and schizophrenia.

4. **Symptoms of withdrawal patient**

    The gross interference with the function of personality is shown in motor behaviour, intellectual activity and emotional responses.

(i) Motor behaviour

    Motor behaviour may show complete indifference to surroundings. Patient may be content to sit alone and day-dream. Posturing may express primitive or sexual wishes. Behaviour may show an active resistance to any form of suggestions. There may be periods of overactivity.

(ii) Emotional responses

Emotional responses may be inadequate, apathetic; patient may show extreme tension through a sudden burst of overactivity. The patient may show his reactions in combination or in sequence or may show one type of reaction consistently.

(iii) Intellectual disorders

Autistic fantasy ideas may be fused, resulting in neologism. Thinking may block suddenly. Loss of integration in the intellectual process. Hallucinations and delusion. Auditory and visual hallucination are the most common. There may occur a sudden violent upheaval characterised by silliness, grimacing, posturing, delusion and hallucination.

During the period of stupor the patients maintain rigidity, assume positions and may show waxy flexibility, muteness, etc.

5. Nursing care

One of the most challenging nursing problems that exists is to help back to healthy social participation the patient who has emphatically turned his back on interpersonal relationships and the society in which he lives.

(i) Psychotherapeutic environment

The recovery of a patient with a severe withdrawal pattern of behaviour must be based on reduction of his perception of himself in relation to others. He must be able to see himself as he is, lose his negative attitude towards himself, and rebuild a new perception in its place. Normal society has failed to accomplish this, therefore, a new type of existence, oriented to make possible such re-education, is indicated.

Provide security. Support his opinion consistently. Assist the patient to move towards the reintegration into society. Physical environment can do this in several ways. They are:

(i)   Staff's attitude towards a patient as an individual with a dignity. So patient develops trust in others.

(ii)   The routines should make reasonable expectations of behaviour with the stimulus to which the patient will be exposed offering the opportunity for response.

(iii)   Demands made upon him for response should offer him some degree of success and call for increasingly complex behaviour.

(iv)   The routine should also include some activities preventing stereotyped performance.

(v)   Attention to reality is important.

(vi)   Keep the physical setup clean, cheerful to provide stimulation on a pleasant level of reality.

(vii)   If the patient's withdrawal is an active form of rejection, the environment should be restricted to permit tactful observation and to limit the possibilities of destructiveness towards others or self.

(viii) Keep his social disability in mind and provide group and community oriented work.

(ii) Interpersonal relationship

Healthy interpersonal relationship cannot be establis at once. From the beginning an attempt can be made to build rapport on a foundation that will lend itself to healthy growth by the patient. Make consistent, steady attempt to draw the patient into some response, without at the same time, demanding a specific response. The patient must be left free to respond without retaliation for the patient's failure to respond. When a patient responds, do not have a high expectation about his social skills. But acknowledge his response with tolerance.

The verbal communication of the patient also poses problems. He uses the language in a highly personal way and has his own individual meaning for words, phrases and sentences. Seek out the patient to communicate your interest in him. Sitting quietly beside a patient saying nothing for brief but consistent periods conveys its message.

It is wise not to get trapped in the patient's intellectual fantasies, not to argue about them, and not to attempt to reason them away. Do not sanction his behaviour.

Careless personal exposure, indiscriminate defecation and carelessness in regard to personal appearance and odors tend to arouse strong disapproval. They are marks of regression. Express quiet acceptance without prudishness.

Constantly make attempts to build the patient's badly shattered opinion of himself. Encouragement and praise may be used, but only when they are justified and can be accepted by the patient. The sensitive ego of the patient must be nourished carefully.

(iii) Physical needs

Care must be provided for the personal appearance and personal cleanliness of the patient. The patient may need assistance for his nutrition, excretion and exercise. Observation of symptoms of physical illness is important.

Help him to take a bath, brush his teeth, comb his hair, shave, etc. Do these things for him in the beginning, getting his help as much as possible. Give supportive comments and sincere praise, when he has done it. Keep the routine simple and consistent, so that he will not have to make a decision. Simple behaviour modification techniques may be used, e.g. reinforcing with extra food privileges.

If the patient is in catatonic stupor, he may have to start on tube feedings and gradually work upto normal feeding. Provide meals and supervise while eating. Find out the likes and dislikes of the person before this illness and serve the food, keeping that in mind. Offer drinks of juice or milk between meals.

(iv) Protection

Certain protective needs of patients with withdrawal patterns grow out of their particular symptom syndrome. Sudden attacks on others, often without any evident personal animosity, can occur, as well as sudden jumps or wall-diving that may result in personal injury or death.

Because of their indifference to social standards exhibited through exposure, profanity or crude sexual gestures, they need to be isolated from the group. They are also in need of physical and psychological protection from others in the environment who are more aggressive. Patients need to be protected from idleness and unbridled indulgence in fantasy.

Prevention of suicidal attempts could be another problem in some withdrawn patients. The precautions to prevent suicide, as discussed earlier, have to be adopted here.

(v) Group relations

Passively withdrawn patients can hold group interactions with depressive patients, while actively withdrawn patients can completely disrupt a group. In group relations, the withdrawn patient is always in danger of attack from more aggressive patients. Encourage and support the withdrawn patients to participate in socialised activities. To begin with, the patient may be placed with one or two similar patients. ater he may be placed in a larger group containing more active members. The members of the group should remain fairly constant. Assign him to do simple tasks which he can do independently, later shared activities can be asked to be done. Encourage the patient to express himself non-verbally (through writing, drawing). Interact with him on a one-to-one basis initially, then help him progress to small groups, and to larger groups as tolerated.

(vi) Convalescence

Withdrawn patients need reassurance with regard to his return to society. He can be encouraged to talk through his feelings about going home. Socialised activities should be encouraged, and the patient should be given opportunities to develop social skills. Arrange for the patient to go out for shopping, picnics and entertainment. Help him in doing shopping, taking bus and coming back. If it is a house-wife some planning and retraining on domestic skills are necessary. Help him/ her to get involved with social groups outside. Help him/ her to make plans as to what he is going to do with self in future.

II Mania

Manic behaviour is characterised by an increased activity level and by an "elevated expansive or irritable mood".

Manic behaviour often occurs in bipolar affective disorder (previously known as manic-depressive psychoses) which is characterised by a history of high and low moods with periods of relatively normal and effective functioning in between.

Mania is a part of affective disorder. It is opposite to depression. Here mood is elated with an increase in the quantity and speed of physical and mental activity. In 1882, Kahlbaum described mania and melancholia as stages in a single disease process. Emil Kraepelin (1899) introduced the term 'manic depressive psychosis'.

Manic episodes usually come with depression. Then it is called bipolar disorder. When it occurs in single

327

episodes, it is called as manic episodes. Most of these disorders tend to be recurrent. Often such episodes are related to stressful situations.

1. Definition

Mania reflects elevation of mood, increased activity and self-important ideas.

According to ICD-10, the core features of mania are:

(i)   Elevated mood; almost uncontrollable excitement.

(ii) Increased psychomotor activity; eg. pressure of speech, irritability.

(iii) Increased self-esteem and grandiose.

2. Etiology

D.S.M. III R (Diagnostic Statistical Manuals Revised in 1987) states that bipolar disorder appears to be equally common in men and women.

The onset of illness is between 15-25 years. The mean age of onset is 30 years. Frequently it has been seen that in manic phase of illness patient abuses alcohol.

Predisposing factors

(i)   Biological theories

(a)   **Genetics** : Studies indicate that there is an increased incidence of bipolar disorder in first degree relatives of individuals with the disorder than in the general population.

(b) **Biochemical :** In depression, there is an in dication of lowered level of norepinophrine during episodes. Opposite appears to be true of an individual experiencing a manic episode.

It is also been suggested that manic individuals have a lower intracellular sodium distribution during episode.

(ii) **Psychological theories**

(a) **Early childhood experiences :** Maternal dep-rivation, prolonged absence of a parent.

(b) **Sociological :** Life events, e.g. death, marriage, financial loss, etc., environmental stress, chronic conditions.

(c) **Behavioural :** Koplan and Sadock says that when depression subsides, the ego may still be too weak to control the impulsive excessive behaviour dominated by the id. In otherwords, mania is a defense against depression.

3. Classification

According to ICD-10, mania is classified according to the severity of illness.

(i) **Hypomania :** This is a lesser degree of mania. There is a mild elevation of mood, increased activity and energy. But not severe enough to disrupt work or social rejection. Symptoms are present for at least several days.

(ii)   Mania without psychotic symptoms :
Here symptoms are severe enough to disrupt
ordinary work and social activity. Mood is
irritable and suspicious.

(iii) Mania with psychotic symptoms : It is
a more severe form of mania. Grandiose ideas
may develop into delusions like delusion
of identity, persecution and self-neglect.

(iv) Manic episodes, unspecified

4.   Clinical features

(i)   Elevated, expansive or irritable mood

The elevated mood can pass through the following
four stages, depending on the se verity of manic episode.

(a)   Euphoria (mild elevation of mood) :
Increased sense of psychological well-being
and hap-piness not in keeping with ongoing
events. This is seen in hypomania (Stage I).

(b)   Elation (moderate elevation of mood) :
Feeling of confidence and enjoyment along
with increased psychomotor activity. This
is classical of mania (Stage II).

(c)   Exaltation (severe elevation of mood) :
In tense elation with delusions of grandeur.
Seen in severe mania (Stage III).

(d)   Ectasy (very severe elevation of mood) : Intense
sense of rapture or blissfulness. Seen
in delirious or stuporous mania (Stage IV).

Along with these variations in elevation of mood, expansive mood may be present, which is increasing and unselective enthusiasm for interacting with people and surrounding environment.

At times, elevated mood may not be apparent; instead, irritable mood may be predominant, especially when the person is stopped from doing what he wants.

(ii) Thought process

(a) **Flight of ideas** continuous rapid shift from one topic to another.

(b) **Pressure of speech** is so forceful and strong and difficult to interrupt.

(c) **delusions of grandeur** individual believes that he or she is all-powerful, possesses feeling of greatness.

(d) **Delusion of persecution** individual believes that someone desires to harm him.

(iii) Motor activity

There is increased psychomotor activity ranging from overactiveness and restlessness to manic excitement where the person is 'on-the-toe-on-the-go', (that is, involved in ceaseless activity). This activity is usually goal-oriented and based on external environmental cues.

(iv) Other features

Sleep is usually reduced with a decreased need for sleep.

Appetite may be increased but later there is usually decreased food intake, owing to marked overactivity.

Insight into the illness is absent.

Sexual desires are increased.

Decreased attention and concentration.

Easily distracted by slightest stimulus.

5. Diagnosis

Diagnosis is made by proper history taking and mental status examination after finding positive criteria of mania. Episodes should last for at least a week.

6. Medical management

(i) Hospitalisation

Usually manic patients require admission when delirious mania is present, accompanied with financial losses, loss of career or family disintegration.

(ii) Drugs

Antipsychotic drugs - chlorpramazine (30-800 mg) Haloperidol, (1-100 mg), Triflupramazine (2-40 mg)

These drugs bring the symptoms of acute mania under rapid control. Doses are gradually increased.

Antipsychotics blocks the post-synaptic dopamine receptors in the basal ganglia, limbic system, etc.

Lithium is used in the prevention and treatment of manic episodes.

Dosage for acute mania   – 1800-2000 mg

For maintenance   – 300-1200 mg

Therapeutic serum level   – 0.7-1.2 mEq/L

For prophylasis   – 0.4-0.8 mEq/L

Lithium carbonate reduces both relapses and recurrences. Therefore, it is important that for prophylaxis lithium should be continued for at least a year or longer. Lithium elimination should be carried out every six weeks.

Carbamazepine is useful in acute mania and prophylaxis of bipolar and unipolar disorder.

(iii) Electroconvulsive therapy (ECT)

Those manic patients who cannot tolerate drugs or where drugs are contra indicated ECT is the choice. For those who do not respond to conventional drugs, E.C.T. is mandatory.

7. Nursing care

(a) Milieu management

It is an important dimension of the nursing care of the manic patient because manic patients test the ward perhaps more than any other group of patients.

Manic patients have tendency to create conflict, pick on vulnerable persons (patients and staff), blame others, test limits, and shift responsibility to others.

Nursing staff must use consistency in their approach, and all the staff must be aware of intervention strategies and should not fall prey on the statement of the patient, like "you're the only one who understands".

Since manic patients are hyperactive, talkative, irritable and angry, it is important to decrease environmental stimuli. Since the patient is distractible and responds to all sorts of environmental cues, it is important to modify his environment as much as possible. Helpful environmental modifications include a private (if possible) quiet room; limited activities with others; scheduled rest periods; gross motor activities, for example, walking, sweeping to discharge some of his need to be active; and a public room free from a blaring TV or stereo.

Manic patients can become hostile and aggressive. It is important for the staff to deal with this aggressiveness in a calm, confident manner. If the patient is escalating, an antipsychotic drug such as haloperidol can be administered to prevent physical aggressiveness, and potential weapons (e.g. chairs) can be removed. Limits and the consequences of violating those limits should be reviewed.

Since manic patients lose their appetite and are too 'busy' to eat, it is the nursing staff's responsibility to ensure that they are adequately nourished. The following are several useful techniques for helping the patient to maintain body weight.

- Provide the patient with foods that can be eaten on the 'run' (finger foods). Some patients cannot sit for a long time to eat.

- Provide high-protein, high-calorie snacks for the patient. A vitamin supplement may be indicated.

- Weigh the patient regularly. (Sometimes daily weights are needed).

Manic patients also experience insomnia. The nurse can help the patient maximise the opportunity for sleep by:

- Providing a quiet place to sleep

- Structuring the patient's day so that there are fewer stimulating activities towards bed time.

- Not allowing caffeinated drinks and provid ing warm milk before bed time.

- Assessing the amount of rest the patient is receiving. Manic patients are not capable of judging their need for rest, and exhaustion and deaths have resulted from lack of rest.

8. Some guidelines to work with manic patients

(i) Establish rapport and build a trusted relationship.

● Show acceptance of the patient as a person.

● Use a firm, yet calm, relaxed approach.

● Make only those promises you can realistically keep.

● Prevent the patient from harming self or others.

● Provide a safe environment to the patient.

(ii) Decrease disorientation, hallucination, delusions bizarre behaviour, dress, sexual acting out.

● Reorient the patient to person, place and time as indicated (call the patient by name,

335

tell the patient your name, tell the patient where he or she is, the date, etc.)

- Spend time with the patient.

- Ignore or withdraw attention from bizarre dress, behaviour, and sexual acting out as much as possible.

- Set and maintain limits on behaviour that is destructive or adversely affects other patients.

- Help the patient to recognise delusions. Never convey to him that you accept the delusions as reality. Directly interject doubt regarding delusions as soon as the patient seems ready to accept this. Do not argue with the patient but do present a factual account of the situation as you see it.

Attempt to discuss the delusional thoughts as a problem in the patient's life. Ask if the patient can see that the delusions interfere with his or her life.

- Interpret the patient's pattern of hallucinations. Be aware of all surrounding stimuli including sounds from other rooms (such as television or stereo in adjacent areas).

Try to decrease stimuli or move the patient to another area.

Avoid conveying to the patient the belief that hallucinations are real. Do not converse with the "voices" or otherwise reinforce the patient's belief in the hallucination as reality.

(iii) Decrease hyperactivity, restlessness and agitation.

- Decrease environmental stimuli whenever possible. Respond to cues of increased restlessness or agitation by removing stimuli and perhaps isolating the patient.

- Limit group activities in terms of size of group and frequency of activities based on the patient's level of tolerance.

(iv) Promote rest and sleep.

(v) Encourage nutritious diet.

(vi) Provide emotional support.

(vii) Promote compliance with lithium carbonate therapy.

Questions

1. What do you mean by 'withdrawn behaviour'?

2. Explain the psychodynamics of withdrawn behaviour.

3. Discuss the characteristics of withdrawn patient.

4. List down the symptoms seen in withdrawal patients.

5 How will you take care of a patient who is withdrawn?

6 What is mania?

7. How does ICD-10 define mania?

8. What are the causes of mania?

9. How do you classify mania?

10. Identify the clinical features of manic patients.

11. What are the medical managements for manic patients?

12. Describe the role of nurses in taking care of patients who are diagnosed as mania.

Prevention of accidents amongst the mentally ill

Any situation or a set of unforeseen circumstances which needs immediate intervention amongst mentally ill becomes the major responsibility of nurses in psychiatric wards.

Any stress-induced factor leads to pathologic response that physically endangers the affected individual or others, or significantly disrupts the functional equilibrium of the individual or his/her environment, and calls for immediate intervention.

Accidents among mentally ill patients constitute one of most significant health hazard in our country. An insurance company estimated that 80% of all major accidents are due to personality factors. Some studies have been made to rule out environmental and other causative factors involved in accident. The findings report that the disturbed mental state of the patients, such as extreme confusion or grave depression, leads to accidents.

An accident is commonly defined as an event which happens by chance, or is unexpected or unfortunate. In other words accidents are accidental.

Various physical events in the patient life may require immediate action. Some of these may occur frequently in the psychiatric hospital than elsewhere. Such situation includes - burns, scalds, fractures, sprains, accidents, self-inflicted wounds, choking, poisoning, sudden unconsciousness and so on. Therefore the nurse's task is to be very alert and attentive, causation in caring of mentally ill patient.

1. Accidents outside the hospital

(i) Psychological factors

Many studies have suggested that motor accidents involve a higher incidence of such characteristics as emotional instability, impulsiveness, lack of alertness, egocentricity, irritability, inadequacy, and poor social and vocational adjustment.

Psychoanalytic observations have stressed the significance of such precipitating factors as:

- inadequate or incomplete repression.
- unconscious need for punishment.
- strong repressed motives.

(ii) Psycho-physiological factors

Most important is the role of toxic factors such as barbiturates, antihistamine, marijuana. Alcohol studies indicate that people are more susceptible to accident when they have been taking tranquillisers or sedative drugs. And also when they are suffering from extreme fatigue.

II Dynamics of accident susceptibility

The ability to avoid accidents depends on a number of complex psychological and psycho-physiological processes. The individual must maintain an attitude of constant alertness to the external world. An ability to evaluate possible risk situations, together with the capacity to act quickly and intelligently to avoid them, and finally the wish – conscious or unconscious – to avoid such a situation. Anything that interferes with any of these processes, even temporarily, will increase the individual's accident susceptibility. Physiological influences such as fatigue, alcohol and sedative drugs may impair a person's efficiency. Similarly, emotional influences lead to accidents. Whenever a person is temporarily tensed and angry, unusually elated or preoccupied with worries, his capacity to deal with risk situations are impaired. More so, the mentally ill who have cognitive impairment affective disturbances prone to accidents.

III Management

(i) Psychotherapy is indicated where chronic, unconscious, motivational factors appears to be involved.

(ii) Education to the patient's to create awareness of risk, inappropriate responses in risk situations, etc.

(iii) Correction of personality through behaviour therapy.

IV Accidents within the psychiatric setup

(i) Unauthorised departures

Very frequently it is noticed in a ward setup that the patient is found to be missing from ward. Therefore it is necessary for ward nurses to keep an eye on patients, e.g., during meal time. The nurse should also explain this to the relatives of risk patients in order to have a constant watch on the patient.

If a patient is found to be missing, an immediate report must be submitted to the senior staff or psychiatrist in charge. Accurate reporting can greately simplify the task and even prevent any tragedy. The nurse should be able to report where the patient was last seen and by whom.

(ii) Prevention of self harm or punishment

Often accidents are the result of emotional turmoil. Patients with hostility, depression, withdrawal, alcoholism, usually require a close watch since they express their negative feelings particularly the hostility, and tend to turn it inward upon themselves. Instead of punishing themselves with their feelings by depression, they punish themselves with physical wound. Therefore it is mandatory for nurses to develop trust with the patient.

Positive reinforcement with small accomplishment and encouragement of the patient to ventilate his feeling would bring the accidental events under control.

(iii) Prevention of suicide

Patients with schizophrenia, severe depression and alcoholism are more prone to suicidal risks. The care of patients with suicidal risk has been dealt with earlier.

(iv) Prevention of mechanical injuries

Possibilities of mechanical injuries, electrical mishaps, burns, poisoning and infection are present even in a psychiatric setup.

Smooth, even floors, fixed floor coverings and well-lighted rooms help prevent falls which cause most mechanical injuries. Patients must be warned when floors are wet, and movable objects kept out of passage way.

Proper positioning of patients while sitting in bed, wheel chair or chair and sufficient support to maintain position is necessary, especially for elderly weak patients.

342

Side rails on bed should always be used if there is a possibility of patient rolling out of bed. It is mandatory for a patient who is seriously ill, elderly, unconscious, or having post-ECT unconsciousness, intoxication, etc.

Areas in which the patient may walk should be dry and free of obstacles and slipping hazards. Night lighting should be provided in the patient's rooms and corridors and in bathrooms and toilets.

All toilet, bath and shower facilities should be equipped with grab bars to provide assistance for ambulatory patients. Time to time checking and repairing of those articles used for shifting the patients like a trolley for post-ECT patients, a wheel chair for an alcoholic withdrawal patient - will also prevent accident.

(v) Protection from electrical hazards

Psychiatric patients are more susceptible to electrical hazards than normal individual. Unsafe handling of electrical equipment can cause even death to a patient.

Electricity may damage the body in four ways:

a) It affects the nervous system.

b) It affects the heart by causing ventricular fibrillation.

c) Electric current in contact with the skin may scorch and coagulate tissue.

d) Electricity causes muscles to contract causing intense pain.

(vi) Protection from fire

Most of the fire accidents are due to carelessness.

Early detection, prevention of spread and extinguishing of the fire are important. Each hospital has a general policy. Nurse should know where to phone, what to report. The entire hospital staff should be familiar with measures for fire prevention and control.

Allowing the patients to smoke inside the ward becomes the source of fire accidents amongst mentally ill. Keeping a room aside for smoking and allowing the patients to smoke would prevent fire accident.

(vii) Protection from nosocomial infection

Although most psychiatric patients are admitted with their psychological problems, still there are chances of getting many systemic infections because of their negligence of personal hygiene and poor hygienic practice.

Further, it is wise to use disposable syringes and needles and they need to be carefully discarded. This will prevent HIV (Human Immuno deficiency Virus) infection from a positive patient to others. Multiple drug addicts, alcoholics who have the poor intake need to be protected from infections as their resistance power is low.

Inspite of constant efforts taken to prevent accidents amongst mentally ill, there are patients who require psychiatric first aid. Their illness bring threat to their survival. Nurse's observations in the behavioural changes of the patient can predict the emergencies and prevent accidents.

Patients with suicidal risk, emotionally distressed – the grief stricken, excitable, overactive, confused, delirious, fearful, paranoid, psychopathic liar, exploiter, aggressive, violent stuporous, panics and impulsive may cause accidents due to their disturbed behaviour.

Attending to their needs in time, anticipating, appreciating and adjusting to dangers with confidence would prevent the accidents. Nurses must know what to do quickly. There are certain principles of nursing psychiatric patients. They are:

1. Observe directly and assess.

2. Supervise unobtrusively by doing things for and with the patients.

3. Practice due care, i.e., take steps to minimise care.

4. Satisfy wants and needs casually as a matter of course.

5. Promote and protect individuality and encourage the patient to talk.

6. Get to know the patients as individuals.

7. Learn how to yield gracefully.

8. Be ready to agree rather than contradict.

9. Learn to anticipate and check as a matter of routine.

10. Reassure and persuade rather than order.

11. Be always ready to listen.

12. Avoid reproach and the use of words with moral overtones.

13. Minimise frustrations and boredom. It prevents patients pushing each other or hitting. Keep them engaged with various activities.

14. Avoid undue fussiness and setting too high a standard.

15. On the first sign of restlessness or change of mood be more watchful.

16. Adjust to dangers with caution and confidence.

Questions

1. Name the commonest accidents that could be formed amongst the mentally ill.

2. What are the factors lead to accidents amongst the mentally ill?

3. How does accident occur in psychiatric hospital?

4. List the basic principles underlying the management of accidents susceptibility of psychiatric patients.

5. How will you prevent accidents in psychiatric hospital?

6. Outline the principles to be followed by nurses to prevent accidents amongst mentally ill.

Observation, reporting and recording

I Observation

Observation is "the gathering of relevant information about the patient's ability to function as an independent person which enables the nurse to formulate nursing intervention consistent with the patient's real needs".

Observation is also defined as "the act of noting and recording facts and events". Observation is not just looking around. But it is characterised by the utilisation of all appropriate sense organs.

Process

The psychiatric observation process can be broken into two main parts:

(i) The nurse's impression of the patient in his clinical environment and information gained from other sources which will be used as a functional comparison.

(ii) The nurse's interview.

A. Nursing impression

It must be emphasised that the observation process is not an exercise in spying on the patient but a mutual activity of involvement. The patient must be made to feel that he is participating in his own care.

Observational elements

1. How does he behave whilst on the ward ?

This is a general impression of the major behavioural presentation and a statement about the physical manifestations of his emotional difficulties and conflicts.

2. How does he respond to his fellow patients?

No person lives in a vacuum. He may withdraw from them, appear to be suspicious of them or to be frightened of them. He may select certain people to sit with and talk to or he may become angry or agitated in the company of others. Who are his friends?

3. How does he respond to the staff?

Are there any particular staff members to whom he seems able to relate? Does he ignore them or seek them out? Does his mood change in their presence?

4. How does he socialise?

How does he behave in set circumstances? Is he withdrawn or does he mix well?

5. What questions does he ask to the staff patients?

This will give a good indication as to what is uppermost in his mind and not what the nursing staff feel he should be thinking.

6. Does he leave the ward?

Where does he go and with whom? How does he seem when he leaves and on his return? Is there anything which occurs on the ward which precedes his departure from it?

7. Is he able to orient himself to his surroundings?

Is he disoriented; if so, how? Does he find his environment a threat? Does he know where to find the toilet, the TV or radio, the lounge, his bed, the kitchen, the nursing station and the dining area?

8. Does he seem interested in himself?

How does he dress? Is he smart or untidy? Does he attend to his personal hygiene? Does he shave or does she wear make-up?

9. Is he dependent or independent?

Does he ask to be helped or does he use other methods of gaining attention which are less acceptable?

10. What is he able to do for himself ?

Does he make his own bed, get his own drinks and serve himself at meal times ?

11. Does he have any physical pain?

Does he complain of pain, biologically identified or otherwise? Does he request pain-killers?

12. Does he eat well?

Does he eat all his meals ; if so, what does he eat? Does he appear to enjoy his food, or is he simply going through the motions? Does he have any particular favourities in his diet?

13. Does he excrete regularly?

Is fluid balance appropriate? Does he experience difficulty in voiding? Is he constipated? Has he any pain or discomfort?

14. Does he sleep well?

The night staff will make comments about his sleep pattern on his first night of admission and use this as a base line for further information. Does he sleep during the day; if so, when?

15. Does he have any physical problems?

Has he any physical handicap that might inhibit him in his bid to be independent. Does he have a walking aid, a hearing aid or spectacles? If so, does he use them? Is he capable of independent mobility?

16. Does he have visitors?

Yes or No? How do the visitors affect him? Is he pleased to see them and does he enjoy their company, or does he become irritable and argumentative? How does he seem when they have departed? Does he discuss the visits?

17. When does he appear most satisfied?

18. Under what circumstances does his behaviour change?

When is he relaxed, disturbed, aggressive, happy, anxious, apprehensive, cheerful, bright or distressed?

19. Does he appear to be a threat to himself or others?

Is he a danger to himself? Does he have self-destructive behaviour? Is he at risk when left alone? Does he threaten others. If so, why, when and whom?

20. How has he changed since admission?

This is an important area because it will indicate the effect of his change of environment. Is he more relaxed and at peace or is he more disturbed and less likely to be able to lead an independent life?

The answers to the above questions form the nucleus of any observational impression made by the nurse. Nurses do not involve asking questions to the patient on a formal basis, but it will be necessary to verify the observations with him, especially if they are causing either distress or disturbance.

The Nurse's interview

The type of interview used will be of a semi-structured nature. Open-ended questions are put to the patient so that he has an adequate opportunity to express himself within a frame work.

Observational criteria

The interview will include those questions not already answered by the nurse's impression. The following constitute the basis for those questions:

1. What does the patient expect from being in the hospital?

2. How does he experience his own illness?

3. Why does he feel that he has been admitted?

4. What are his impressions of his hospitalisation?

5. What does he expect from the nursing staff?

6. What does he feel capable of doing for himself?

7. How do his psychiatric symptoms affect his ability to function as he would wish?

8. Has he any awareness of his condition, situation or behaviour?

9. How does he cope with his activities of daily living?

10. What influence do his relatives or visitors have upon him?

11. What is troubling him most at present?

12. What would he most like to be able to do at present?

13. What influence has the hospitalisation process had upon him?

14. What does he feel his potential for progress and rehabilitation is?

15. How does he see his future?

Factors that affect observation

1. Physical, mental and emotional states, feelings and needs.

2. Cultural, social and philosophical values and background.

3. The senses involved and their functional abilities.

4. Past experiences associated with the present situations and its context.

5. Meaning of the observed event.

6. Interests, preoccupation, preconceptions and motivational level.

7. Tendency to view other's opinions or deas as your own.'

8. Tendency to make judgements on the basis of first impression and then avoiding changing that impression.

9. Prejudice.

10. Favouritism.

11. Knowledge of or familiarity with the situation being observed.

12. Environmental conditions and distractions.

13. Attitude and reactions of others. For eg., even if your perception and observations are accurate, if others do not agree with you, then you are likely to conform to group opinion.

Criteria of observation

(i) Must be purposeful

(ii) Must be planned

(iii)   Must be objective

(iv)   Must be accurate

(v)   Must be complete

(vi)   Must be systematic

Methods of observation

1   Based on time

(i)   Intermittent observation

(ii)   Continuous observation.

2.   Based on technique

(i)   Direct observation (Nurses obtain data by simply watching the patient's behaviour)

(ii)   Indirect observation (includes motion picture, television, videotape or other devices of recording.)

3.   Based on personal involvement

(i)   Participant observation : Nurse actively participates along with patient in some work and collects information.

(ii)   Non-participatory observation : Observing what is happening to the patient and what he feels about it provides the nurse with the basis for her care plans.

II   Reporting

Reporting is a process of giving oral or written account by one member to another in the health team. Probably no other single factor is more vital to good patient care and ward management than prompt, complete reports. No organisation can function effectively and efficiently without a definite system for communication.

1. Definition of a report

Reports are forms of communication prepared by individuals to pass information and understanding from one or more individual to another individual or group (Goddard).

Report is to give an account of something that has been seen, heard, done or considered.

2. Purpose of reports

(i)   To convey factual information.

(ii)   To communicate between the members of the team.

(iii)   To avoid duplication of work.

(iv)   To show the kind and amount of service rendered over a specific period.

(v)   To illustrate progress in reaching goals.

(vi)   To provide basic facts for service and to aid in studying health conditions.

(vii)   To aid in planning.

(viii) To interpret the services to the public and to other interested agencies.

(ix)   To enable the nurse to judge the quality and quantity of work done.

(x)   To help better student education.

3. Criteria of a good report

(i) Reports should be made promptly, if they are to serve their purpose well.

(ii) Even if some information which is urgent in nature had been sent by telephone message, it should be followed by a written report. Eg. serious accidents.

(iii) A good report is clear, concise, complete. It is written with all pertinent information, and identifying data are included - the date and time, the people concerned, the situation, the signature of the person making the report.

(iv) No extraneous material is to be added.

(v) Reports must present facts systematically with logical arrangement and should be well-organised for easy understanding.

(vi) The important information must stand out.

(vii) Reports are clearly expressed and presented in an intersting manner.

4. Types of reports

(i) Oral reports

(ii) Written reports

(iii) Taped reports

(iv) Automated intershift nursing reports

(i) Oral reports

Oral reports are given when the information is for immediate use and not for permanancy. They may be based on material included in a written report. Eg. staff and student nurses give oral reports while changing duties.

(ii) Written reports

Williamson identifies the parts of a written report that, if used synchronised, ensure a well-organised logical presentation. These parts consist of a title, an abstract for quick view of the problem, body and conclusions and recommendations. Such a structure is valuable to the communicator because it exerts discipline that forces rework and refinement and allows for better understanding.

Written reports are made when the information is to be used by several people or is more or less of permanent value. Eg. day and night reports, unusual conditions found in patients which may lead to complaints, etc.

(iii) Taped reports

Taped reports provide help to evaluate the quality of leadership performance of nurses over a period of time and the nursing care given to a group of patients. The taped reports include information on new nursing problems, their attempted solutions and outcomes. Through the use of taped report of morning and evening, the senders and receivers become much more conscious of the need for accurate information.

(iv) Automated intershift nursing reports

Many exploratory studies have been conducted to develop computerised nursing reports in an effort to resolve the problem of getting accurate, consistent, comprehensive reporting of nurse's "observations" and care of patients.

5. Characteristics of a report

(i) Recognition of pertinent factors to report. When to report, to whom to report and how to report.

(ii) Honesty in reporting : include factual data, avoid ambiguity, never manipulate the records and record actual observation rather than opinions.

(iii) Simplicity.

(iv) Adequate information with clear, concise and meaningful terms.

(v) Professional quality : Give reports in intelligible terms, observe good English, utilise proper mechanics of printing or writing. Spell correctly.

(vi) Avoid use of abbreviations except in clinical charting. Be neat and utilise proper signature.

(vii) Legal acceptability.

(viii) Emphasis on constructive and positive factors, that is, those that affect the welfare of all concerned.

(ix) Adherence to the objectives, principles and policies of nursing service.

(x) Written reports should be signed and dated with the position or status of the writer.

(ix) Written report is more comprehensive and may be kept as a permanant record. Oral reports on emergency situations always should be confirmed in writing.

(xii) Statistics are used in a report to convey information as to many facts which may be expressed numerically. Tabular presentation is the form most commonly used and is more practical. Graphs and charts are more pictorial presentations of statistical facts and can be effectively used in annual reports.

(xiii) Reports may also be made on printed or mimeographed forms. The report forms which commonly used in hospitals are daily service report, accidents, transfer and discharge of patients, who are seriously ill and the census of patient in each ward, etc.

6. Varieties of reports in psychiatric hospital

(i) Day and evening report and night report

The purpose of this is to provide the means of transferring pertinent information about patients to the head nurse, the ward evening and night nurses to the nursing office and to the evening and night supervisors.

Only that information which is necessary to give a general picture of the ward need be included such as census, the names, diagnosis and general condition of patients, the patients admitted and discharged.

In psychiatric hospital, nurses are expected to do mental status examination of the patient for acute psychiatric patients every day for a period of 15 days, and alternative day for one month and weekly once for the later period. For chronic psychiatric patients monthly once reviewing physical health and mental status are recommended. Reports of mental status of patients are complied.

The events like suicidal attempts of patients, accidents among the mentally ill, escape of patients from hospital, parole (temporary discharge) of the patients must also to be reported.

The discharge of psychiatric patient through Board of Visitors have to be reported and a written report has to be made.

(ii) Census report

The daily census or the number of patients in the hospital at midnight, furnishes the important source material for hospital statistics. The night nurse completes the ward census, which is collected by the night supervisor and the total hospital census is calculated.

(iii) Inter-departmental reports

Reports of the patient to be discharged are sent to business/account section for the bill settlement; the repairing work of the ward is reported verbally to the engineering section for rectification. Promptness and accuracy are essential if the work of each department has to run smoothly.

(iv) Inter-agency report

A system of inter-agency referral between the hospital and the health and social agencies of the community has been established for the welfare of patients.

Nurses give report of the treatment given to the patient so far in their nurse's notes, doctor writes the present health status of the patient with his referral note to other health agency. It also includes attitude of the patient and his family towards illness, existing social and psychological problem, if any.

(v) Special report on unusual condition in the patient

There are times when a hospital is criticised for what is claimed to be negligence or poor care because of a condition which lead to discomfort and perhaps serious harm to a patient. It is advisable to report any situation which might raise a question relative to the quality of nursing or medical care.

(vi) Reports on mistakes and accidents (legal reports)

As it is needed for the legal purposes, the report should contain the exact hour, the date, the name of the patient, the visitor, or the employee, the name and position of the nurse who made the mistake or witnessed the incident.

(vii) Report on complaints

If the complaint of a patient or visitor is of such serious nature that it cannot be easily resolved by the ward personnel to the satisfaction, it is wise to report it to the nursing office in writing. It must include the statement of complaint, justification for it as seen by the nurse, measures taken to overcome the dissatisfaction, the results, and the name of the people involved. As with all other reports, it is dated and signed.

(viii) Evaluation report

An evaluation report on each nursing staff member is usually required by nursing service when personnel is centrally employed. It should include member's self-evaluation, ward incharge's evaluation, writing of anecdotes by head nurse, the actions taken, the progress made, etc. It should be kept confidential. Every effort should be made to write meaningful reports which will be helpful to nursing service administration and benefit the individual staff.

(ix) Laboratory and other reports

The laboratory tests of various specimens like blood, sputum, urine, stool, cerebrospinal fluid, metabolism, test,

X-rays and other special studies needed in the medical care of a patient. When the service is rendered the findings are recorded on the requisition form which is returned to the nursing units and the reports become the part of patient's record.

(x) Nursing office reports

The chief nursing officer prepares a consolidated report of absentees and sends to billing clerk to deduct the wage from the salary of casual workers; she also prepares monthly postings of nursing staff and the people working under her.

(xi) Annual report

The annual report of department gives an account of the nursing department to the governing body and to the administrator. It provides facts from which to appraise the nursing service. It provides an opportunity for the director of nursing to point out the needs of the nursing department. It provides an opportunity for the director of nursing to acquaint the community with facts concerning the nursing service of the hospital since it is customary to print this report in the annual report of the hospital.

III Recording

Record is that which is written to perpetuate a knowledge of events. They form an administrative tool used to collect and verify information (Goddard).

Record is defined as a written, formal, legal documentation of a client's progress and treatment. It is also defined as a permanent, a long-lasting account of something on film or in writing which can be reproduced.

1. Purpose

1. To provide information.
2. To facilitate vertical and horizontal communicaton.
3. To provide source of reference for research work.
4. To protect administration and supervision against legal entanglement.
5. To serve as a basis for improvement.
6. To provide a means for determining the achievements.

2. Principles

1. It should be for a special purpose.
2. Legal documents should contain true facts.
3. It should be written clearly and legibly.
4. Accuracy and completeness are essential.
5. Wording should be easily understood.
6. Record of interview, mental status exam, etc. have to be written immediately.
7. It should be neat, simple and concise.
8. Provision for easy access and kept safe.
9. The necessary stationary should be available.
10. Records are confidential and to be produced only for legal calling and not to anybody other than the treating team.

Questions

1. Define observation.

2. What are the process involved in psychiatric observation?

3. Explain the elements involved in psychiatric observation.

4. What constitutes the basis for nurse's interview?

5. Discuss the factors affecting observation.

6. Name the criterias of observation.

7. Outline the methods used for observing psychiatric patients.

8. What is reporting?

9. List down the purpose of writing reports.

10. Identify the criterias of good report.

11. How do you classify reports?

12. Enumerate the characteristics of a good report.

13. What are the reports maintained by nurses in psychiatric hospital? Explain the reasons for maintaining them.

14. What is a record?

15. Mention the purposes of recording.

16. What are the principles to be kept in mind, while recording an event that occurred in the psychiatric ward?

Legal aspects of the care of mentally sick patients

Procedure for admission into and discharge from mental hospitals

Law reflects social norms. It is important to know the current law that affects psychiatric nursing practice; if psychiatric nurses know the law, use it effectively and help change it as necessary, the psychiatric patient can receive respectful care and the nurse will be recognised as a knowledgeable professional.

The care and treatment of people who are mentally ill have changed dramatically since Philippe Pinel first crusaded to gain humane conditions for them. Today, the mental health professional is confronted by legislation and court decisions outlining methods and procedures all focused on admission into and discharge from mental hospitals.

The legal aspects of psychiatry in India are based on the Indian Lunacy Act, 1912 (16th March).

It is derived from English Lunacy Act, 1890. It contains 8 chapters.

Chapter I contains the preliminary information and definitions of certain terms used in psychiatric treatment. They are as follows :

i) **Asylum**	:	Means mental hospital for lunatics established or licensed by the Central or any State Government.
ii) **Lunatic**	:	Means an idiot or a person of unsound mind (unsoundness of mind is defectiveness of reasoning, either partially or completely).
iii) **Criminal Lunatic:**	:	Means any person for whose detention in or removal to an asylum, jail or other place of safe custody an order has been made in accordance with the provisions of Section 466 or 471 of the Code of Criminal Procedure 1898 or of Section 30 of Prisoners Act, 1900 (or of Section 103 A of the Indian Army Act, 1911). Criminal lunatic is a person who qualifies to be criminal and is also a lunatic.
iv) **Reception Order**		Means an order made by a magistrate or a police officer in a presidency town (i.e. with commissioner system of police) to detain under the provisions of this act for the reception into an asylum of a lunatic other than a lunatic so found by inquiry.
v) **Relative**	:	Includes any person related by blood, marriage or adoption.
vi) **Medical Officer**	:	Means a gazetted medical officer in the service of the Government and includes a medical practitioner declared by general or special

	order of a State Government to be a medical officer for the purposes of this act.
vii) Medical Practitioner	: Means a holder of a qualification to practice medicine and surgery which can be registered in the United Kingdom in accordance with the law for the time being in force for the registration of medical practitioners and includes any person declared by general or special order of a State Government to be a medical practitioner for the purposes of this act.
viii) Cost maintenance	In an asylum includes the cost of lodging, maintenance, clothing, medi-cine and care of a lunatic and any expenditure incurred in removing such a lunatic to and from an asylum.

Chapter II contains mainly the procedure to be followed to admit a psychiatric patient into a mental hospital and discharge him from mental hospital.

According to this act, no person can be detained in an asylum except when he is a criminal lunatic or is found so on inquiry or has come with reception order.

Procedure for admission into a mental hospital

(a) Voluntary admission

According to Indian Lunacy Act, the admission may be voluntary i.e. any person who is a major (above 18 years of age) can go to the asylum and apply in writing for admission. Then the Medical Superintendent or Incharge, with the consent of at least 2 members of board of visitors can admit the patient. The visitors are appointed by the State government. There are usually 3 visitors (minimum) for each mental hospital, of which one will be a general practitioner and one will be the I.G. of prisons.

(b) Reception order on petition :
admission through a magistrate

Reception order is issued by a magistrate or a police officer in the presidency town for the detention of a lunatic in an asylum. There should be:

(i) Petition in writing by a relative (guardian, parent, wife, husband, etc.). A relative of the patient can submit a petition to a magistrate for a reception order for admission into the mental hospital. The petitioner must be a major and must have personally seen the patient within 14 days of making the petition. The petition has to be on a special form giving all particulars of the patient and has to be supported by two medical certificates, written on separate papers.

Each medical certificate shall state the facts upon which the person certifying has formed his opinion that the alleged lunatic is a lunatic, distinguishing facts observed by himself from facts communicated by others (and no reception order on petition shall be made upon a certificate founded only upon facts communicated by others). These should be from 2 medical men, one should be at least a medical officer. The other certificate can be from any registered medical practitioner. Both the medical men must have examined the patient independently within 7 days of submitting the application. In other words, these days of submitting the application. In other words, these 2 certificates should not be more than 7 days old and the petitioner should have seen the patient within 14 days.

The certificates should categorically state that the patient is "a lunatic and a proper person to be taken charge of and detained under care and treatment and this must be based on facts observed during medical examination. Each medical certificate is a legal document and therefore, the medical practitioner must be very careful to give a certificate to avoid legal complications. The patient can ask for examination by other two medical people and sue for damages if he is wrongfully certified. So whenever a medical certificate is given for certification, the medical practitioner must be convinced that certification is advisable and possible.

The magistrate will make a decision either with or without making an enquiry or personally examining the patient. If he is satisfied, he will issue a reception order, after getting consent from the petitioner in writing that he would meet the cost of maintenance of the patient in the mental hospital.

(c) **Reception order not on petition :**
admission through police

Any police officer in charge of a police station can arrest any person whom he believes to be a wandering or a dangerous lunatic, or a lunatic who is neglected or cruelly treated. Police officers have been empowered to detain such patients only for 24 hours and then produce them before the Magistrate. After examining the lunatic, if the Magistrate concurs, he issues a reception order. If he doubts, he can get the lunatic medically examined.

369

The Magistrate can detain the patient for 30 days but not in continuity (he issues 3 reception orders of 10 days each). The Magistrate can direct the guardian to bear the expenses. The state Government can be asked to bear the expenses if there is no one around to look after the patient and patient is a problem.

In case of the cruelly treated, the Magistrate can advise the guardians to look after the patient or otherwise they can be imprisoned for a term (one month) for willful negligence.

No reception order shall be made, save in case of a lunatic who is dangerous and unfit to be at large, unless the Magistrate is satisfied that the person in-charge of an asylum is willing to receive the lunatic and the petitioner or some other person committed in writing to the satisfaction of the Magistrate to pay the cost of maintenance of the lunatic.

No reception order shall continue to have effect after the expiry of thirty days from the date on which it was made unless the lunatic has been admitted to the place mentioned therein within that period.

No Magistrate shall make reception order for the admission of any lunatic into any government asylum outside the state in which the Magistrate exercise jurisdiction (i.e. about sanitation, food and treatment)."

(d) Reception order of criminal lunatics

A criminal lunatic has to be admitted into a mental hospital on the order of the presiding officer of the court. These criminal lunatics can be of 3 types.

(i)   Those who cannot stand the trial because of unsound mind.

(ii) Those who are acquitted because of unsound mind, at the time of committing the crime (e.g. meningitis).

(iii) Those who become lunatic while in prison. The visitors of the mental hospital must visit the criminal lunatics, at least once in 6 months.

An order directing the reception of a criminal lunatic into any asylum which is prescribed for the reception of criminal lunatics shall be sufficient authority for the reception and detention of any person named therein in such asylum or in any other asylum to which he may be lawfully transferred.

(e)   Reception after judicial inquisition

If a person is found lunatic after judicial inquiry, the high court or the district court has the authority to issue a reception order for admission into a mental hospital.

Chapter III briefly describes the procedure to be followed for administering the care, treatment and discharge.

Procedure for discharge from a mental hospital

(i)   In the case of voluntary admission, the patient can ask for a discharge by submitting an application in writing and the superintendent of the mental hospital has to discharge him within 24 hours of receiving the application. Medical superintendent does not have the power to detain the patient and he has to discharge him within 24 hours except if the reception order is in progress in court or inquiry is going on against the patient.

(ii) In cases of patients admitted under reception order on petition, the petitioner has to apply to the superintendent of the hospital who can discharge the patient if he is convinced that the patient is fit to be discharged. Medical superintendent has to obtain consent of Board of Visitors for discharging the patient. Medical superintendent has to give in writing to the petitioner whether he can be discharged or not.

(iii) In the case of a patient who is admitted into a mental hospital by the police, he can be discharged if the family members agree in writing to take proper care of him and if the superintendent or the board of Visitors is convinced that he is fit to be discharged.

(iv) A patient who is admitted after a judicial inquiry can be discharged only after another judicial inquiry.

(v) In the case of criminal lunatics, the superintendent on the advice of the Board of Visitors, will have to recommend to the Government health department. Those who are fit to stand trial will have to be sent to the court. Those who were transferred from the prison will have to be handed over to the prison.

Transfer of lunatics

Transfer of lunatics from one asylum to another in the same state or other shall be with the consent of the State Government (of the state).

Escape and recapture

Every person received into an asylum under any such order as is required by this Act may be detained therein until he is removed or discharged as authorised by law, and in case of escape, may by virtue of such order, be retaken by any police officer or by the person in charge of such asylum. If the lunatic is not a criminal lunatic or against whom a reception order has been made, the power to retake such escaped lunatic under this section shall be exercisable only for a period of one month from the date of his escape. This does not apply to a criminal lunatic, who after cure has to be handed over to the police.

The remaining chapters (IV to VIII) deal with proceedings in Lunacy in Presidency Town, Proceedings in Lunacy Outside Presidency Towns, Establishment of Asylums, Expenses of Lunatics and the Rules to be imposed by the State Government regarding care of lunatics.

Although the majority of the mental hospitals in India observe Indian Lunacy Act of 1912, there are few states that have adopted Indian Mental Health Act 1987.

Indian Mental Health Act is derived from Mental Health Act (22nd May 1987) of England and Wales (1959 amended in 1982). Based on the persistent efforts of Indian Psychiatric Society, the Ministry of Health introduced the Indian Mental Health Bill in the Lok Sabha but before it could be passed, the bill lapsed when the Parliament was dissolved in 1980. Later, the same bill was introduced afresh in 1981. At that time, the Hon'ble Minister of Health, Shri B. Shankaranand introduced the Bill (Bill No. XL1) in Rajya Sabha, and the Bill became an Act in 1987. (Act No 14 of 1987).

The attitude of the society towards persons afflicted with mental illness has changed considerably and it is now realised that no stigma should be attached to such illness as it is curable, particularly, when diagnosed at an early stage. Thus, the mentally ill persons are to be treated like any other sick person and the environment around them should be made as normal as possible.

Mental Health Act 1987 is considered to be necessary:

(i) to regulate admission to psychiatric hospitals or psychiatric nursing homes of mentally ill persons who do not have sufficient understanding to seek treatment on a voluntary basis, and to protect the rights of such persons while being detained;

(ii) to protect society from the presence of mentally ill persons who have become or might become a danger or nuisance to others;

(iii) to protect citizens from being detained in psychiatric hospitals or psychiatric nursing homes without sufficient cause;

(iv) to regulate responsibility for maintenance charges of mentally ill persons who are admitted to psychiatric hospitals or psychiatric nursing homes.

(v) to provide facilities for establishing guardianship or custody of mentally ill persons who are incapable of managing their own affairs.

(vi) to provide for the establishment of a Central Authority and State Authorities for mental health services.

(vii) to regulate the powers of the Government for establishing, licensing and controlling psychiatric hospitals and psychiatric nursing homes for mentally ill persons.

(viii) to provide for legal aid to mentally ill persons at state expense in certain cases.

Critique of the Mental Health Act, 1987

The Mental Health Act contains 10 chapters. Chapter I deals with preliminary informations and definitions of the terms. Few of these are: "

Mentally ill person : (the term lunatic deleted) A person who is in need of treatment by reason of any mental disorder other than mental retardation."

Mental ill prisoner : A mentally ill person for whom detention in, or removal to, a psychiatric hospital, psychiatric nursing home, jail or other place of safe custody, by an order referred to in Section 30 has been made."

Psychiatric hospital or psychiatric nursing home

A hospital or, as the case may be, nursing home established or maintained by the Government or any other person for the treatment and care of mentally ill persons includes a convalescent home established or maintained by the Government or any other person for such mentally ill persons. (But does not include any general hospital or general nursing home). The term "lunatic Asylum" term is being replaced by Psychiatric hospital or Psychiatric nursing home).

Psychiatrist : A medical practitioner possessing a post-graduate degree or diploma in Psychiatry recognised by the Medical Council of India, constituted under the Indian Medical Council, 1956.

Reception order : means an order made under the provisions of this Act for the admission and detention of a medically ill person in a psychiatric hospital or psychiatric nursing home.

Temporary treatment order : A temporary treatment order passed by a Magistrate under Sections 20 or 21.

Chapter II describes the provision for establishing mental health authorities at centre and state level. These authorities will regulate, develop, direct and coordinate the Mental Health Services under the Central Government. They will advise the government on mental health matters. They supervise the psychiatric hospitals and psychiatric nursing homes and other mental health agencies. They also have the jurisdiction to renew or cancel the licenses.

Chapter III deals with the establishment of psychiatric hospitals and psychiatric nursing homes. It gives the ample scope for establishing separate psychiatric hospitals for children, addicts, psychopaths and mentally ill persons.

Chapter IV contains the new procedures for admission and detention of patients in a psychiatric hospital or psychiatric nursing home. It has some very progressive concepts. In it, the procedure for admission of psychiatric patients has been simplified.

Under the new Act, it is not the Board of the Visitors but the medical officer in charge of the hospital who can admit such a patient on a request, even without any application made by a patient. Similarly, the person so admitted can be discharged within 24 hours. This simplification of the procedure would bring the admission procedure of psychiatric patients at par with other patients suffering from physical illnesses.

(a) Admission on voluntary basis

Major : Application on a prescribed form by any major to the medical officer in charge of the hospital or nursing home for admission has to be accepted. If the medical officer in charge is satisfied that he needs treatment, such a person can be admitted. (This is done on the discretion of the medical officer in charge and not on the will of the patient. No permission is required from Board of Visitors)

Minor : The nearest guardian can apply for admission on a prescribed form. If a minor attains majority, an application by the inmate has to be made within 1 month for continuation of inpatient treatment or the patient will be discharged.

Admission under special circumstances

Part II of the Chapter IV brings out an entirely new concept and a novel procedure of 'admission under special circumstances'. This will help in admitting any mentally ill patient who does not or is unable to express his/her willingness for admission as a voluntary patient. Such a patient may be admitted and kept as an in-patient in a psychiatric hospital or psychiatric nursing home, on an application made in his/her behalf by a relative or a friend of the mentally ill person, if the medical officer in charge is satisfied that it is necessary to do so in the interest of the mentally ill person.

The patients admitted under this clause cannot be admitted for a period exceeding ninety days except in accordance with the other provisions of this Act or the reception order should be obtained. This procedure will help in admitting patients who are non-cooperative or unwilling to give consent without going to a Magistrate, provided such a mentally ill person is examined either by two medical officers working in a hospital or nursing home (one should be a gazetted medical officer) or is accompanied by two medical certificates from outside.

If the relative thinks that the medical officer in charge is misusing the Act, he can apply to the Magistrate of the area, who issues a notice to the relative who got admitted the patient in the hospital. If he is satisfied, the patient may be discharged.

Part III of the Chapter IV deals mainly with procedures on reception orders made on the application by relatives of the patient. It also incorporates a new provision authorising the medical officer in charge of a psychiatric hospital or psychiatric nursing home to keep a voluntary patient, or a patient admitted under special circumstances, for a longer period in the patient's interest. However, the basic procedures regarding reception orders on production of mentally ill persons before a Magistrate remain unchanged in this section.

The Act states like this, for admission under reception order,

378

i) On application : The relative (husband, wife, nearest guardian or friend) can apply to the Magistrate in writing supported by 2 medical certificates (one from a gazetted medical officer) for admission of a mentally ill patient. No person who is a minor or has not seen the mentally ill patient within 14 days, shall make an application.

The medical officer in charge, under whose care (hospital or nursing home), the mentally ill patient is undergoing treatment under a temporary treatment order, can give an application to the Magistrate that the in-patient treatment is required to be continued for more than six months.

ii) On production before the Magistrate : The mentally ill patients (making obscene scenes, dangerous to the society, having violent behaviour or cruelly is treated) detained by the police officer are produced before the court within 24 hours.

It should be accompanied by 2 medical certificates. Then the Magistrate may issue a reception order. The relative who willfully neglect the patient may be punishable with fine which may extend to one thousand rupees.

Admission in emergencies

If the mentally ill patient is in danger and the medical officer in charge thinks so, then such type of patients may be admitted. But within 72 hours, the patient should be produced before the Magistrate or if he cannot be shifted, the Magistrate is asked to come to the psychiatric hospital or the psychiatric nursing home and get the patient examined and pass a reception order. These 72 hours are exclusive of the examination period. If the Magistrate cannot come, it is the jurisdiction of the Magistrate to extend the time period (72 hours).

Temporary treatment order

It is issued by the Magistrate of the area. It is done in such cases who are admitted when there is a risk to the person's own life or to that of others.

If medical officer in charge feels that it is necessary to bring the legal authorities into picture, he can apply to the Magistrate or the relatives can go to the Magistrate to get an order issued for treatment. Only one medical certificate is required. This order (from the court) is valid for 6 months.

Miscellaneous admissions

There is provision for admitting the mentally ill patient on humanitarian grounds (e.g. wanderers) or they can be admitted for observation. The social workers come and take the patients to the Magistrate to obtain an order pending report by medical officer.

Chapter V of the Act deals with **Inspection, Discharge, Leave or Absence and Removal of Mentally Ill Persons.**

Unlike the provisions in the old Indian Lunacy Act, the new Act insists on inclusion of psychiatrists and social workers as members of Visitors' Board. It also gives a clear direction in respect of the working of Visitors Board. Under the new Act, the visitors will have no role in the admission and discharge of a mentally ill patient. The visitors shall not be entitled to inspect any personal record of an in-patient which in the opinion of the medical officer in charge are confidential in nature.

One of the major problems faced at present by all mental hospitals is that many visitors never attend any meeting and still they remain members of the Visitors Board. The new Act contains a provision to cease the office of such a visitor from the Board, if he does not participate in the joint inspection for three consecutive months. At the same time, the Act also makes it mandatory on the part of psychiatrist in charge of a case to examine at least once in every three months, a patient detained in jail under the various provisions of the Act.

The Mental Health Act states in the following manner about functioning of Visitors Board :

The State Government shall appoint for every psychiatric hospital and psychiatric nursing home in the state, not less than five visitors of whom at least one shall be a medical officer, preferably a psychiatrist.

The Director General of Health Services shall be the exofficio Chairman of Board of Visitors. For mental health offenders I.G. Police is also exofficio Chairman.

At least one medical officer (as per Indian Medical Act, 1956) is required in the team, preferably a psychiatrist. The other members, would have an aptitude and exposure to mental health problems.

Board of Visitors should visit the hospital at least once a month and at least 3 members of the team should be present. The Director General of Health Services should visit once in 6 months.

Whenever the Board of Visitors visit the hospital, they should write remarks in the visitors book about the working of the hospital.

Every person who is detained in jail shall be visited at least once in every three months by a psychiatrist, or if a psychiatrist is not available, by a medical officer.

Discharge

Part II of Chapter V deals with procedures for discharge of any person on the recommendations of two medical practitioners, one of whom shall preferably be a psychiatrist. There is also a provision in this section for the discharge of a mentally ill patient on application made by a patient so detained, or on an undertaking by relatives or friends.

The Mental Health Act describes the discharge procedure of mentally ill person in the following ways:

Discharged procedure for those who seeked voluntary admission

When the patient desires for discharge, he shall apply in writing. If the patient does not want but the medical officer in charge feels that the patient may be discharged the medical officer in charge writes to the Magistrate who then issues an order for discharge. If the patient does not follow, then there is provision for penalty.

If the patient can obtain 2 medical certificates other than those by which he is admitted, leave of absence may be granted for 60 days (if the need arises).

The application for leave of absence should be accompanied by a bond, with or without sureties for such amount as to take proper care of the mentally ill person, to prevent the mentally ill person from causing injury to himself or to others and to bring back the mentally ill person to the psychiatric hospital or nursing home. The leave of absence may be granted by the medical officer in charge but total duration of leave of absence may not exceed 60 days.

Any mentally ill person (other than a voluntary patient) may be transferred from one psychiatric hospital or psychiatric nursing home to another in the same state or other state with the consent of the Government of that state.

Part III of Chapter V deals with the leave of absence which gives a further scope of flexibility in admission and discharge of patients admitted under reception order and makes the system more flexible.

Part IV of Chapter V deals with safeguarding and removal of mentally ill persons from one psychiatric hospital to another. It also includes provisions regarding admission, detention and readmission in certain cases.

Judicial safe guards for patient's rights

Chapter VI deals with judicial inquiry regarding alleged mentally ill persons possessing property, custody of his person and management of his property. It incorporates some newer provisions which are consistent with other civil laws and procedures governing management of such property by managers.

There are more safeguards now for the patients and there is a greater penalty for misuse of the property by the managers, etc.

The Mental Health Act states in the following manner:

- The inquiry of the mentally ill person (on the request of a relative or public curator, Advocate General) is done by the legal or police authorities. Inquiry may be required when the patient is

- produced before the magistrate by the police officer.

- admitted under special circumstances (when a relative feels that the act is misused)

- in case of emergencies when the Magistrate is not satisfied that the patient is an emergency case and he is acting to avoid criminal responsibility.

In case of miscellaneous admissions,

If the admission is done for vested interests, then the Magistrate before issuing a reception order, orders for an inquiry:

– the district court may appoint a guardian for the mentally ill person and for management of property when it is satisfied that the mentally ill person is not fit to look after himself. Every manager, within a period of six months from the date of his appointment, gives an inventory of the immovable property belonging to the mentally ill person. The manager cannot lease out or sell any immovable property of the mentally ill person without the permission of the court. Every manager gives an account of the property and assets in his charge within three months of the close of the financial year.

These appointments may cease once the District court is satisfied that the mental illness has ceased.

Humanitarian provisions

Chapter VIII contains a very novel and explicit provision for protection of human rights of mentally ill persons.

It emphasis that:

– No mentally ill person shall be subjected during treatment to any indignity (whether physical or mental) or cruelty.

– A mentally ill person under treatment shall not be subjected to mechanical restraint, solitary confinement or other harsh measures unless the medical practitioner concerned is satisfied that there are compelling circumstances which justify resort to any such measure (the medical practitioner has to note down in such cases).

– No mentally ill person under treatment shall be used for the purposes of research unless such research is of direct benefit to him for purposes of diagnosis or treatment or such person being a voluntary person has given his consent in writing or the guardians of the minors have given consent in writing.

- No letters or communication sent by or to a mentally ill person under treatment shall be intercepted, detained or destroyed.

Penalties and procedures

Chapter IX deals broadly with penalties and procedures for establishment or maintenance of psychiatric hospitals or psychiatric nursing homes in contravention of the various clauses under the Act. It also makes the penalties relatively more severe and explicit.

Miscellaneous

Chapter X deals with some miscellaneous items and clarifies certain procedures and explanations, followed by the medical officer in charge of the hospital. He has to prepare the report of modus operandi of hospital every 6 months and send it to the authorities. In case he fails to do this, he can be charged with inefficiency for not doing his duties properly.

The medical Officer in charge is responsible for the supply of all requisites (food, sanitation etc.) to the psychiatric hospital or psychiatric nursing home.

The Mental Health Act represents not only an attempt to introduce the latest concepts and knowledge in the field of mental health, but also incorporates the growing demands and aspirations of the people to get better facilities with less rigid and irksome procedures relating to admission and discharge of psychiatric patients. There is also a conscious effort to demystify mental illness and treat it at par with other physical ailments. Similarly, the present legislation gives more emphasis on looking after the interest of psychiatric patients, and their well-being. It is far ahead of similar provisions in other developed countries.

Questions

1. What are the procedures used to admit and discharge a patient in mental hospital as per Indian Lunacy Act 1912?"

2. How does admission and discharge procedure differ between Mental Health Act 1987 and Indian Lunacy Act 1912.

3. Define the following terms :
   i) Asylum·
   ii) Reception order
   iii) Lunatic
   iv) Board of visitors
   v) Leave of absence

4. Write short notes on :
   i) Voluntary admission
   ii) Admission through reception order.
   iii) Importance of implementing Mental Health Act 1987.
   iv) Admission on emergencies.
   v) Judicial safeguards for patient's rights.

———

387